D0451574

ARE YOU A VICTIM?

- Do you feel tired all the time?
- Do you have to have coffee, cola, or alcohol to get you through the day?
- Are you forgetful, indecisive, irritable?
- Do you suffer from insomnia, depression, headaches, trembling, drowsiness, crying spells, cold sweats, mental confusion, anxiety, dizziness, indigestion, allergies, obesity, craving for sweets, lack of sexual energy?

YOU MAY BE SUFFERING FROM HYPOGLYCEMIA—

one of the world's most frequently misdiagnosed diseases!

Dr. Paavo Airola, internationally recognized nutritionist and leading exponent of biological medicine, explains in this book what hypoglycemia is, how to know whether you have it, and how a simple, common-sense approach can completely eliminate symptoms of this "hidden" disease.

By the Same Author:

HOW TO GET WELL
ARE YOU CONFUSED
REJUVENATION SECRETS FROM AROUND
  THE WORLD—THAT "WORK"
HOW TO KEEP SLIM, HEALTHY AND YOUNG
  WITH JUICE FASTING
CANCER: CAUSES, PREVENTION AND
  TREATMENT—THE TOTAL APPROACH
SWEDISH BEAUTY SECRETS
STOP HAIR LOSS
SEX AND NUTRITION
HEALTH SECRETS FROM EUROPE
THERE *IS* A CURE FOR ARTHRITIS
HYPOGLYCEMIA: A BETTER APPROACH
THE MIRACLE OF GARLIC
EVERYWOMAN'S BOOK

Books by Paavo Airola are available at
all better health food stores and book stores.

SEE BACK COVER OF THIS BOOK
FOR DESCRIPTION AND PRICES

HYPOGLYCEMIA:
A BETTER APPROACH

by PAAVO AIROLA, N.D., Ph.D.

Introduction by J. P. Hutchins, M.D.

MEDICAL EDITORS,
CONTRIBUTORS, AND
ADVISORS

Gabriel K. Cousens, M.D.
Bill Gray, M.D.
J. P. Hutchins, M.D.
Michael B. Schachter, M.D.
David Sheinkin, M.D.

HEALTH PLUS, Publishers, Phoenix, Arizona, 1977

Copyright © 1977 by
Paavo O. Airola

All rights reserved. No part of this book may be reproduced in any form or by any means, without permission in writing from the publisher.

ISBN 0-932090-01-X

First printing, February 1977
Second printing, August 1977
Third printing, May 1978
Fourth printing, October 1978
Fifth printing, May 1979
Sixth printing, September 1979
Seventh printing, January 1980
Eighth printing, July 1980
Ninth printing, July 1981

Published by
HEALTH PLUS, Publishers
P.O. Box 22001, Phoenix, Arizona 85028

Printed in the United States of America

To the millions of victims of hypoglycemia —the insidious and devastating disease of civilization—who suffer needlessly, misdiagnosed, mistreated, and unaware that simple, safe, and effective means of correcting their condition and restoring health are available;

and to the growing number of open-minded and dedicated doctors who, for the benefit of their patients, have the courage to use new, unorthodox therapeutic approaches —even if they happen to be contrary to established medical thinking and practices—

I dedicate this book.

Paavo Airola, Ph.D.

ACKNOWLEDGEMENTS

I wish to express my sincerest thanks to Bill Gray, M.D., Gabriel K. Cousens, M.D., Michael B. Schachter, M.D., and David Sheinkin, M.D., for their valuable contribution to this book; these doctors have used my hypoglycemia diet extensively in their practice and report on their experiences in Chapter 11.

My special thanks to J. P. Hutchins, M.D., for his unselfish contribution and assistance in proofreading and editing the manuscript before publication, for writing the Introduction, and for his invaluable expert advice.

Last, but not least, I wish to thank Anastasia for her editorial, artistic, and secretarial assistance in preparation of this work—help as much appreciated as it was needed—as well as for being a source of inspiration and encouragement.

TABLE OF CONTENTS

INTRODUCTION

by J. P. Hutchins, M.D.

Dr. Hutchins is the vice-president of the International Academy of Biological Medicine; the past president of the International Academy of Applied Nutrition; a member of the American Academy of Medical Preventics; and a member of the American College of Metabology. He is one of the leading practitioners of biological medicine in the United States, using nutrition, acupuncture, herbology, osteopathy, homeopathy, and other wholistic approaches to healing. He is a nationally recognized lecturer and an authority on nutrition and has appeared on numerous T.V. and radio programs. Dr. J. P. Hutchins practices in Wilmington, California.

Hypoglycemia is a "new" but an increasingly common affliction. Although our medical establishment continues to claim it does not exist, those of us in active practice know better. Many patients who are mistakenly diagnosed as schizophrenics, neurotics, psychotics, alcoholics, or mentally disturbed, are actually suffering from the low-blood-sugar syndrome. Their health problems are often miraculously solved by simple dietary changes.

Dr. Airola's new book, *Hypoglycemia: A Better Approach,* is an important contribution to the betterment of health, not only in this country, but around the world. It will revolutionize the treatment of hypoglycemia—the devastating and incapacitating disease which is spreading like an epidemic. The Airola Diet, which is the essence of his unique approach to the management of hypoglycemia, is not only able to control the symptoms of low blood sugar, but actually can help to cure the condition and restore health. I have been personally and professionally associated with Dr. Paavo Airola and his work for many years, and have used his diet and his ideas in the treatment of my hypoglycemia patients. As a rule, they respond almost immediately to the Airola Diet and their symptoms disappear. The importance of this book, therefore, cannot be overestimated.

Dr. Airola has done a superb job of writing a clear, simple, yet comprehensive book on a very difficult subject. He precisely and succinctly defines hypoglycemia, explains how you can tell if you have it, and offers detailed programs that are easy to understand and follow. I recommend this book highly, not only for those who suffer from hypoglycemia, and for all serious students of nutrition, but also for all of my fellow physicians, researchers, nutritionists, herbologists, homeopaths, osteopaths, naturopaths, chiropractors, acupuncturists, and all those who are interested in a wholistic approach to healing.

I predict that this epoch-making book will be translated into many languages and will undoubtedly be used as a textbook in medical schools. This is the first truly authoritative book on hypoglycemia. In my opinion, Dr. Paavo Airola is the foremost nutritionist in the world today—in the depth and scope of his knowledge. He is also a leading authority on biological medicine and wholistic approach to health and healing. This background has enabled him to write a well-documented and well-researched text that no other nutritionist or physician has had the time or know-how to produce.

We are all indebted to Dr. Paavo Airola for writing this revolutionary book. His unique hypoglycemia treatment will prevent much misery and suffering and change the lives of many who are plagued by constant fatigue, insomnia, irritability, depression, confusion, anxiety, overweight, physical and mental distress, and a sense of futility, giving them hope of complete recovery and living normal, healthy, and happy lives.

This book will also be an indispensable tool in the hands of physicians, helping to decipher the mysteries of this complex, and "hidden" disease, and helping them to take better care of their hypoglycemic patients. On the basis of my own experience, I can attest to the fact that Dr. Airola's approach to the treatment of hypoglycemia is, indeed, as the title suggest, a *BETTER APPROACH*—better than the conventional high-protein therapy, being safer for the patients and bringing more permanent results.

J. P. Hutchins, M.D.

Complexities of Hypoglycemia

Hypoglycemia is the most perplexing, mysterious, complicated, contradictory, as well as controversial and complex "disease" I know. How did I arrive at such a disheartening conclusion? Consider this:

1. The medical establishment—AMA and the affiliated groups, clinics, as well as official medical journals—insists that hypoglycemia is virtually a non-existent condition invented by self-diagnosing health faddists; a popular "in" disease among jet-set high-stress, heavy-drinking hypochondriacs; a new invention replacing ulcers as the status disorder. A famous Mayo Clinic doctor and syndicated medical columnist, Walter Alvarez, M.D., summed up the official view saying, "I have never seen a case of functional hypoglycemia in thirty years of practice." The American Dietetic Association, the American Diabetes Association, and the Endocrine Society joined the American Medical Association in publishing in their official journals strongly worded position statements indicating that hypoglycemia is an *extremely* rare condition.

Yet, such prominent doctors and practioners as Harvey M. Ross, M.D., Robert C. Atkins, M.D., E. M. Abrahamson, M.D., Stephen Gyland, M.D.,

Clement G. Martin, M.D., Sam E. Roberts, M.D. and Alan H. Nitler, M.D., to name a few, consider hypoglycemia to be one of the most prevalent ailments in modern society, a virtual epidemic of major proportions. Dr. Atkins, for example, says that "the commonest condition I am called upon to treat in my practice of internal medicine is low blood sugar (hypoglycemia)."[1] Dr. Cheraskin claims that "the sugar-laden American diet has led to a national epidemic of hypoglycemia."[2] And, Dr. Harvey Ross says that "hypoglycemia has been estimated to affect 10 per cent of the United States population."[3] That's over 20 million people!

2. Some doctors consider hypoglycemia to be a serious, incapacitating *disease*, a contributing factor to such killers as heart disease and even cancer. Others dismiss it as a rather harmless "stress adaptation syndrome", a carbohydrate metabolism disorder that is easily controlled and/or avoided.

3. According to some doctors, the medical definition of hypoglycemia is very simple: too little sugar in the blood, or low blood sugar. They also define hypoglycemia as "the opposite of diabetes" (which is too much sugar in the blood). The offered cure is equally simple: more of easily-available sugar in the diet. Other experts violently oppose this simplistic view of hypoglycemia, claiming that the underlying causes leading to low blood sugar are so complex and so different with each individual that it is almost impossible to find a common therapeutic approach applicable to more than one case.

4. The experts' opinions on correct diagnostic procedures are just as contradictory. While many practitioners feel that a 5 or 6-hour glucose tolerance test (GTT) is a perfectly reliable and conclusive way to

diagnose the condition, others feel that such a test is not only harmful, but also constitutes a very misleading, as well as undependable, way to find the presence of hypoglycemia. The standard medical practice is to consider levels of blood sugar lower than 60 to 80 mg. per 100 ml. as hypoglycemia. But one of the nutrition experts with wide experience in hypoglycemia, Dr. Carlton Fredericks, claims that "there is no number, no point, no range of blood sugar which constitutes hypoglycemia."[4] He says that it is not *how low* the blood sugar level goes, but the *speed* at which it drops that causes the symptoms of hypoglycemia—and only in *some* people, at that!

Are you beginning to be perplexed and confused? Can you see now why I referred to hypoglycemia as the most complicated, mysterious and complex health problem that I know?

But whether or not the experts agree on the definition, classification, diagnosis, or treatment of the hypoglycemia syndrome, your distress and suffering, if you are afflicted with it, is just as severe. You are probably reading this book because you are searching and looking for relief. Because the major hypoglycemic symptoms are mental confusion, emotional instability, low energy level, and neurotic, even psychotic behavior, the condition of hypoglycemia has a serious effect on a person's whole life, including his marital and family relationships; it has, in other words, enormous personal as well as social implications. J. I. Rodale believed that many accidents, family quarrels, suicides, and even crimes are committed by individuals when their sugar levels are pathologically low.[5] Hypoglycemia is, indeed, one of the most devastating ailments of modern man.

Because I have seen so many unhappy, distressed, and miserable individuals whose lives have been wrecked—virtually destroyed—by hypoglycemia, I have decided to write this book to try to help those who are already afflicted, as well as those who may be subjected to this danger in the future. This task is not easy. Although I have authored ten books, one of which, HOW TO GET WELL, outlines successful biological and nutritional treatments for over 60 of our most common diseases and is used as a textbook in several universities, colleges, and medical schools, I feel apprehension as well as a great sense of responsibility as I approach this "simple" problem of hypoglycemia. I can truthfully say that of all the medical problems and ailments that I have studied and researched, this is the most complex, misunderstood, and controversial condition of which I can think.

My work with hypoglycemia and with the research of the causes and effective biological treatments of hypoglycemia began many years ago. I was attracted by the fact that although the controversy and the confusion as to its causes is massive, all experts agree on the most important issue of all —the treatment. The high protein-low carbohydrate diet, the so-called Seale Harris diet, is a universally accepted, endorsed and prescribed diet for hypoglycemia. However, on the basis of my life-long research in nutrition, preventive as well as therapeutic, I am well aware that a high-protein diet, especially on a prolonged basis, can be extremely harmful and may lead to many serious biochemical and metabolic disorders; it may contribute to the development of such serious diseases as arthritis, cardiovascular disorders, osteoporosis, periodontal disease, and even cancer. Therefore, I became naturally very apprensive when I saw thousands of hypoglycemics put on high-animal-protein diets by their physicians. I just could not see the wisdom of trying to control (and that's all the conventional high-protein diet purports to do) the symptoms of an although serious, nevertheless, non-fatal disorder with a diet that I knew would invariably lead to much more serious, possibly fatal diseases.

This led me to interviews with many physicians who specialized in treating hypoglycemia, as well as with hypoglycemic patients who were placed on high-protein diets. Some doctors were displeased with the standard treatment. They have found that although a high-protein diet did control the symptoms of hypoglycemia, their patients complained of feeling tired, being toxic, and developing constipation, arthritis, gout, headaches, and skin disorders. A common complaint of patients on high-protein diets was physical and mental sluggishness, or lack of energy.

Consequently, I developed a new, safer and more effective, dietary program for the treatment of hypoglycemia. First, I encouraged a few doctors to try it on their patients. The response was most gratifying. Several physicians switched from the traditional high-protein diet to my low protein-high natural carbohydrate diet. When the new diet appeared in 1974 as a part of my book, HOW TO GET WELL, many hypoglycemics tried it and I received a great number of letters stating how, with the help of my nutritional program, their health was restored and their low blood sugar conditions were corrected. Then, in 1976, I published a two-part article, *Hypoglycemia: Causes, Prevention, and Treatment,* in Let's Live Magazine's department on biological medicine. Again, the mail from those who tried my diet was overwhelmingly positive. Finally, in the summer of 1976, I conducted three professional seminars for physicians in the United States, describing to the doctors the new approach to the treatment of hypoglycemia. Many doctors started using my diet immediately. In Chapter 11 you will find the reports of some of these doctors on the successful application of my therapeutic program for hypoglycemia with many actual case histories described in detail. In Chapter 12, you will find several letters from those who tried this dietary approach on their own. The general response from doctors and patients was so positive that it convinced me of the necessity for making known to more people this new and better approach to the treatment of this widespread and devastating malady. The birth of this book was motivated by such conviction.

Doctors and hypoglycemia sufferers who tried the new therapeutic approach to low blood sugar as described in this book, agree that it is better than the conventional high-protein approach because it not only controls the symptoms of hypoglycemia effectively, but it actually helps to correct the condition and eventually facilitates a complete restoration of health. The conventional diets, while also able to control the symptoms, are so harmful to the general health of the patients that they actually create even more serious disorders and diseases than those they are attempting to cure. A classic example of the "cure being worse than the disease."

Please note that the nutritional and biological approach to the treatment of hypoglycemia—diet, specific vitamins and supplements, herbs, and other modalities—as reported on the following pages, is not offered as a cure, but as a supportive means of assisting your body's own inherent healing forces by eliminating the underlying causes of disease and thus creating the most favorable conditions for the body's healing power to bring about the actual cure. In other words, the proposed diet and other natural therapies are aimed at helping your body to heal itself. Every individual's response to specific foods, vitamins, and other treatments is extremely different, depending on his specific condition, including: individual nutritional requirements and needs, age, health stature, inherited weaknesses, ability to assimilate nutrients, emotional health, the level of environmental stresses, etc., etc. Since this is the case, I wish to suggest that the information in this book be used in cooperation with a nutritionally-oriented doctor who is trained in both the diagnosis and the treatment of hypoglycemia and who is capable of supervising the progression of the treatment. Although the proposed diet and other programs are simple and self-explanatory, it is never wise to be your own diagnostician and your own doctor. If, after reading this book, you feel that my approach to the treatment of hypoglycemia makes common and academic sense to you, I suggest you take this book to your doctor and abide by his decision regarding the advisability of using the suggested therapies for your specific condition. If your doctor is not familiar with my dietary approach, or if he is antagonistic toward it—and many high-protein oriented doctors still are!—you may write to the publishers of this book and request a list of doctors who are trained to use my approach. The publishers will send such a list on request if you enclose a stamped, long, self-addressed envelope.

Now, let us try to decipher the mysteries and the complexities of hypoglycemia—the insidious and tragic disorder that affects over 20 million Americans, but is almost unknown in most other countries. The proper understanding of the underlying causes and the physiological mechanics of this disease, as well as the proper knowledge of how to prevent and correct it, may give us clues as to why so many of us also suffer from heart attacks, allergies, peptic ulcers, obesity, chronic fatigue, and cancer. Such knowledge may also give us clues as to why so many of us become schizophrenics, alcoholics, tobacco-coffee-coke-drug-addicts, and suicide victims. And we may find out why crime, apathy, moral decay, divorce, family disintegration, and personal and collective irresponsibility are on the increase. You see, chronic low blood sugar, or hypoglycemia, may be at the root of much of the above.

2

What is Hypoglycemia

Hypoglycemia, translated into lay terms, simply means low blood sugar. *Hypo* means low; *glycemia* means sugar. Diabetes is the opposite: high blood sugar, or hyperglycemia. The two conditions, although diametrically opposed, are closely related. Both are caused by the body's inability to use sugar effectively. This is, of course, an oversimplification. And I will admit, right at the onset, that we will have to use a lot of generalizations and oversimplifications—many more than I would like—when trying to define and explain such a complex condition as the hypoglycemia syndrome. This is because, more than any other disease, hypoglycemia and its symptoms, as well as its underlying causes, varies with almost every individual patient. In fact, trying to explain hypoglycemia, especially to a lay reader, seems almost futile. I wish I could skip the whole area and get right to the part of the book that really matters— the part where I can tell you that you don't have to suffer from the hypoglycemia syndrome, that although we do not know exactly how it develops in every case, we do know how we can successfully control its symptoms and even help to correct the condition permanently and restore health.

But, since it would probably be helpful in the effective application of the corrective measures that will follow, I will attempt to give you a short resumé of what we do know, or think that we know, as to the possible causes of hypoglycemia.

Sugar metabolism

Hypoglycemia was officially "discovered" by Dr. Seale Harris in 1924. He was first to describe the presence of abnormally low blood sugar levels and the distinctly defined symptoms that accompany them. The condition was at first called *hyperinsulinism,* and it was considered to be caused by too much insulin in the blood. Excessive insulin burned more sugar than was necessary and caused an excessive drop in the blood sugar level. In diabetes, too little insulin is produced, which results in too much sugar staying in the bloodstream for too long. Thus, in simple terms, an over-active pancreas (where insulin is produced) is blamed for low blood sugar. But the real question is: why is the pancreas overactive?

Thus, both diabetes and hypoglycemia are linked to defective sugar metabolism in the body. What is sugar metabolism and what causes its derangement?

To get answers to these questions, we must understand the relationship and the difference between nutrition and metabolism. Nutrition is related to the foods and liquids that enter our bodies; nutrition science is a study of the nutritional and therapeutic value of foods. Metabolism refers to what happens to the nutrients *after* they enter the body, how they are assimilated, absorbed, utilized, and burned up, and how they are used in various processes involved in keeping tissues and organs well.

The three basic nutrients obtained through foods are carbohydrates, fats and proteins (plus, of course, vitamins, minerals, trace elements, enzymes, etc.). Almost all foods contain all of them, but in varying proportions. The basic human diet, especially as it had evolved since the advent of agriculture, was largely made up of natural complex carbohydrate foods, such as grains, seeds, nuts, vegetables, fruits, and some dairy products. Meat and fish were common only on some parts of the planet and only in small amounts. Our metabolisms, then, were adjusted—genetically programmed to effectively sustain health and prevent disease— to a low protein, low fat, and high natural carbohydrate diet. Even now, in those parts of the world where civilization and industrialization have not yet made their destructive assault, and where the traditional diets have remained the same, the people are free from disease and they enjoy optimum vitality and long life. Their diet is a low protein, low fat, high natural carbohydrate diet (as in Hunza, Abkhasia, Vilcabamba, and Yucatan).

But in the past few hundred years, with the advent of industrialization and the increased wealth that followed it, man's diet has undergone dramatic changes. Meat, fish, and fowl, consumed earlier only occasionally, now have become central to the diet. Concentrated carbohydrates, such as sugar and refined flour, completely non-existent before, now are eaten in increased quantities, reaching an incredible yearly intake of 125 lbs. of sugar and an equal amount of white flour per person in America today! The human metabolic system was not designed to function efficiently and trouble-free on such a diet. The excess of protein and fat, and especially the huge amount of refined carbohydrates, has overloaded our metabolisms and contributed to the long line of diseases directly related to faulty nutrition. Hypoglycemia is but one of these nutrition-related disorders.

Sugar is the fuel our body uses for heat and energy. Normally, sugar is obtained from carbohydrate-rich foods, such as grains, vegetables, potatoes, fruits, bread, beans and corn. The complex carbohydrates are slowly broken down from their long-chain molecules and changed into smaller molecules of absorbable sugar, called *glucose,* which is ultimately absorbed slowly through the wall of the small intestine. This sugar is then carried to the liver, where it is converted into *glycogen* and stored. As the need for sugar arises (remember, sugar is needed for all muscle actions, and especially for brain and nerve function), the stored glycogen is reconverted into a usable form, glucose, and transported by the blood to the areas where it is needed. Thus, when we eat sugar in the form of natural carbohydrates, our blood and tissues usually contain only the amount of sugar needed for their normal function. But when we eat food with refined, white, commercially produced sugar, the small-molecule carbohydrates of these foods are absorbed quickly—sometimes almost instantaneously through the membranes of the mouth and stomach—causing a sudden flood of glucose into the bloodstream. Such a flood of excess sugar into the bloodstream causes a tremendous strain on the pancreas and liver, as well as on the adrenals and other endocrine glands that are involved in regulating blood sugar levels.

Our bodies are well equipped to handle an occasional strain in the form of an excess of ingested sugar. The pancreas produces insulin which is released into the bloodstream where it destroys the excess sugar. But, if we continuously abuse our metabolism by dumping in huge amounts of easily absorbable sugar, the strain on the sugar-regulating organs will be too great. It may damage them to the extent that they will not be able to cope with the continuous insult. Often, the reaction of these organs, especially the pancreas, becomes abnormal (such as an over-reacting pancreas which produces large amounts of sugar-reducing insulin although only an insignificant amount of refined sugar was consumed) resulting in the symptoms of hypoglycemia. And if the pancreas is over-reactive and produces too much insulin, the sugar level in the blood drops abnormally low, depriving the brain and nervous system of much needed oxygen and causing an array of unpleasant hypoglycemic symptoms. Eating sugar in such a situation will not help. On the contrary, it will only trigger the over-responsive pancreas to produce more insulin and make the situation and symptoms worse.

The abnormal reaction or malfunction of the sugar level regulating organs can be caused by other factors of which we will speak later. These other factors include emotional and physical stresses, alcohol, coffee, smoking, nutritional deficiencies, overeating and drugs. But faulty eating habits, especially the excess of refined carbohydrates in the diet, is the factor that contributes most to the development of hypoglycemia.

"I don't eat sugar"

In my consulting work, I often encounter patients with diagnosed functional hypoglycemia who say, "I haven't eaten sugar for years—I never touch the stuff!—how could I have hypoglycemia?"

So few people realize that sugar is concealed in many foods. You may eat an occasional piece of apple pie á lá mode. Did you know that it contains 18 teaspoons of sugar? You drink a glass of orange juice. Did you know that orange juice is 13 per cent sugar? A plain doughnut contains 4 teaspoons of sugar! A bottle of Coca-Cola contains over 4 teaspoons of sugar. Many commonly used sauces, jellies, custards, and canned fruits or juices contain added sugar. It is almost impossible today not to get huge amounts of sugar if you buy your food at the regular supermarket. Virtually all man-made, canned, processed, frozen, or packaged foods contain some form of sugar additive. All commercially sold bread, for example, contains sugar or syrup.

One of the things that many health-oriented people, those who do not eat sugar in any form, do not realize is that they often overload their system with easily assimilable sugar by eating too many sweet fruits, especially dried fruits, such as dates, figs, prunes or raisins. Even without added sugar, these fruits contain so much naturally concentrated sugar that it can easily overtax the pancreas and trigger its over-reaction.

Even worse, the current fashion among many well-meaning health food advocates is to drink excessive amounts of sweet fruit or vegetable juices, such as grape, apple, or carrot juice. This practice can have a disastrous effect on sugar metabolism and can contribute to the development of hypoglycemia as well as diabetes. We all subscribe to the idea of eating whole natural foods. We object to sugar and white flour on the grounds that they are refined, fragmented, concentrated substances. At the same time we gulp huge amounts of juices on a regular daily basis without realizing that juices are not whole and natural foods. They are also fragmented, isolated, concentrated, sugar-laden liquids which our bodies and our metabolisms are not equipped nor programmed to handle. I have seen some people who drink half a gallon, sometimes even a full gallon, of carrot juice a day. Not only do the palms of their hands turn yellow, but a large amount of sugar in this highly concentrated food puts a very real strain on the liver and pancreas. Our bodies are designed to handle foods that are *eaten*. When we eat carrots or grapes, chewing them thoroughly, the carbohydrates and sugars in these foods are gradually and slowly digested and absorbed, supplying an even flow of sugar. But when we drink sweet juices, an excessive amount of sugar that doesn't need an elaborate digestion, but is absorbed quickly through the membranes of the stomach and even the mouth, is suddenly flooding the bloodstream with the demanding strain on the pancreas and liver to quickly neutralize it and restore proper sugar levels. There is a certain maximum level of dietary sugar that our organs can handle without damage. This level was set by maximum sugar that can be obtained by *eating* foods. It has been determined during thousands of years of metabolic and genetic adaptation to the natural environment.

There is another factor to consider regarding the practice of copious juice drinking. Juices are extremely alkalizing foods, containing large amounts of highly alkaline minerals, especially potassium. Juices do have a rightful place and play a very important role in practically every therapeutic program, especially during fasting when they help cleanse and de-acidify tissues affected by acidosis (excessive meat-eating, among other things, leads to over-acidity). However, if juices are used in large amounts, on a prolonged basis, by relatively healthy people, they tend to alkalinize the body too much and cause a condition known as alkalosis. This, again, puts an extra strain on the adrenal glands which must synthesize large amounts of special adrenal-cortical hormone to restore and maintain a normal pH in the body. Most readers are probably aware of the fact that an overly-acid system (too many grains and/or too much meat in the diet) is not a desirable condition and may lead to metabolic disorders, contributing specifically to the development of arthritis and rheumatic diseases. But an overly-alkaline body (too many alkalizing vegetables and fruits, especially in concentrated juice form) is just as undesirable. It may make the body susceptible to many metabolic disorders, especially digestive and assimilative problems as well as an increased susceptibility to infections. Not too acid, but not too alkaline either, is the ideal—pH should be about 6.4 on a urine test, which means slightly acid. Neutral pH is considered to be 7.0.

Now, after this warning about the indiscriminate drinking of sweet juices, especially by hypoglycemics or those prone to hypoglycemia or diabetes, I must hurry to clarify myself before I am misunderstood or misquoted. I am against the *excessive drinking* of juices. Generally, foods should be *eaten,* not drunk. A small amount of juice, 2–3 oz. at a time, can be taken, either diluted 50-50 with water one hour before a meal, or undiluted with meals, provided it is not drunk, but sipped slowly, and salivated well—as any other food. In the treatment of disease, especially during juice fasting, juices are indispensable. (For information about how to use juices therapeutically and what juices to use for specific conditions, please refer to my book, HOW TO KEEP SLIM, HEALTHY, AND YOUNG WITH JUICE FASTING.[6]) Please note, however, that juice fasting, although an essential part of the standard biological treatment of almost every disease, is not recommended for the treatment of hypoglycemia nor diabetes except when prescribed and supervised by an experienced doctor. (Malignancies and active tuberculosis are other conditions where fasting is not advisable.)

The mechanics of hypoglycemia

In summary, the mechanics of hypoglycemia are as follows:

- Dietary starches, carbohydrates, and sugars (many different forms of natural sugars such as sucrose, fructose, maltose, lactose, etc.) are broken down in the process of digestion and processed into glucose.

- Glucose is then changed into glycogen and is stored in this form in the liver.

- Glucose is involved in many vital body processes: it is an energy and heat source, and it is a carrier of oxygen into every cell, especially to the heart, to the nerves, and to the brain. The glucose is needed every second of your life and is constantly released by the liver in proper amounts to meet the need and to assure a healthy functioning of all the tissues and organs.

- Since the dietary sugar first enters the bloodstream before it is picked up by the liver, the level of sugar in the blood would vary dangerously unless controlled by some mechanism. There are several effective mechanisms in the body that keep sugar in the blood at needed levels at any given time.

- If the sugar level is too high, or rises too fast, the islets of Langerhans (the insulin-producing part of the pancreas) produce a hormone, insulin, and send it to the bloodstream. The insulin converts the sugar into other elements and normalizes the blood sugar level.

- If the sugar level is too low, the brain will, through the pituitary and thyroid glands, send a message to the adrenal glands, which then release a different hormone, adrenalin, which will instruct the liver to release some more glucose into the blood.

Ideally, when all these glands and organs function as they should, blood sugar is kept at normal levels. Even if we occasionally abuse our bodies by dietary indiscretions, these sugar-controlling mechanisms are able to cope with the extra strain. But they have their limits! Like any other mechanisms, either within the human body or in man-made machinery, they can break down. When they do, conditions such as hypoglycemia and/or diabetes will result. When sugar gets abnormally high and the damaged pancreas is unable to produce enough insulin to bring sugar down and maintain the ideal balance of glucose in the blood—*it is diabetes.* When sugar gets too low, either because of an over-reactive pancreas that produces too much sugar-destroying insulin, or possibly because of a pancreas under-active in terms of producing the hormone, *glucagon*—an anti-insulin factor which is a controlling substance that blocks the action of insulin when needed—*it is hypoglycemia.*

Now, I must again remind you of the great complexity in the physiology and mechanics of hypoglycemia. There are many, many reasons and causes that may lead to the malfunction and/or breakdown of the whole sugar-controlling mechanism. Causes include not only a simple excess of refined sugar in the diet, nor pancreatic or adrenal underactivity or overactivity, but also such factors as:

- Imbalances in secretions of hormones by other endocrine glands, especially by the pituitary and thyroid.[7]

- Excessive use of alcohol, tobacco, and coffee or caffeine-containing soft drinks.[2,8]

- Systematic overeating, especially of refined carbohydrates and excessive animal proteins.[9]

- Allergies.

- Severe emotional stresses that can cause both the rise and fall of sugar levels, as well as the overexhaustion of adrenal glands which are so essential to proper sugar metabolism. Although our bodies are able to meet the demands of stress at times of emergency, i.e., occasionally, they are not equipped to withstand *constant* stress. The emergency mechanism is set to give a quick response to temporary crises. When crisis or stress, especially emotional stress, becomes permanent, as is often the case in our competitive stress-laden society, the alarm mechanism becomes overtaxed, breaks down, and degenerative diseases result.[7] Hypoglycemia is one of the classic examples of the degenerative processes caused by nutritional abuses, constant stresses, and a generally health-destroying mode of living.

The above-mentioned description and definition of hypoglycemia refers to so-called *functional* hypoglycemia, or hypoglycemia caused by an overactive or oversensitized pancreas, but without a diagnosable pathological development or structural damage. An overwhelming majority of all cases of low blood sugar are functional hypoglycemia. There are, however, other kinds of hypoglycemia, usually referred to as hyperinsulinism. Tumors of the pancreas, benign or malignant, when located in the insulin-producing area of the pancreas, the islets of Langerhans, can result in hyper-insulinism, or excessive insulin production. If these tumors are non-malignant, they usually respond to a hypoglycemic diet as recommended in this book; if they are malignant, a special therapeutic cancer program and even sometimes surgery is necessary to correct the condition. The other cause of hyperinsulinism is an enlargement in the whole insulin-producing area of the pancreas. A defective liver or diseased or malfunctioning pituitary or adrenal glands can also result in hyperinsulinism. All the above-mentioned categories of hypoglycemia are classified as *organic* hypoglycemia.

This book deals mainly with functional hypoglycemia which is responsible, perhaps, for 99 per cent of all cases of low blood sugar.

3

Symptoms of Hypoglycemia

Some people—even some doctors, who should know better—dismiss hypoglycemia as a minor disorder blown out of proportion by self-diagnosing hypochondriacs. Some others consider it to be an extremely dangerous and devastating disease that has hit modern civilization like an epidemic plague. In the words of Dr. Harvey Ross, "It is a disease that will not kill you, but may make you wish you were dead."[3] The main reason for such a discrepancy in the evaluation of the seriousness of this condition is the fact that hypoglycemia, as a single disease, is simple enough—it is blood sugar that is lower than normal. But even this is an unreliable way to diagnose hypoglycemia. There are people who have low sugar levels without hypoglycemic symptoms. There are also many persons who can have symptoms of hypoglycemia, even severe ones, while having blood sugar within normal range.

The biggest problem, however, is the fact that practically every symptom of the expansive hypoglycemia syndrome can be caused by other pathological conditions. This is the reason why hypoglycemia is often referred to as a "great mimicker." It can mimic virtually every symptom in a medical book. What this can mean to a desperate patient is eloquently illustrated by the following actual cases.

Gyland case

Paradoxically, Dr. Stephan Gyland was himself a physician. While busy practicing in Flórida, he fell ill. He experienced weakness, dizziness, faintness, unprovoked anxieties, tremors, rapid heartbeat, difficulties with concentration, and memory lapses. Realizing that a physician is his own worst doctor, he consulted a specialist. He was told that there was nothing wrong with him physically, that he was a neurotic, and that all the described symptoms were "in his mind." He also was told that this disqualified him for the practice of medicine.

But Dr. Gyland refused to accept the "all in your head" verdict and consulted another doctor. In his own words, "During three years of severe illness, I was examined by fourteen specialists and three nationally-known clinics . . ."[10] None of these experts or world-famous clinics, which included the Mayo Clinic, ever tested him for hypoglycemia, although one doctor did suspect low blood sugar; this doctor, however, prescribed candy bars, which, of course, would only worsen his condition. Although they could not seem to find anything wrong with him, the specialists did not hesitate to pass authoratively the assortment of such diagnoses as: brain tumor, neurosis, diabetes, and cerebral arteriosclerosis.

Still very ill and unable to work, since none of the suggested treatments were of help, Dr. Gyland was desperately searching for the solution to his problems by reading medical literature, hoping to find some clues. He happened to see the original paper on low blood sugar and its symptoms, published by Seale Harris, M.D.[11] The symptoms described by Dr. Harris matched Dr. Gyland's in detail! He immediately took the test for low blood sugar which confirmed the diagnosis of hypoglycemia. He went on the hypoglycemia diet suggested by Dr. Harris and *watched his symptoms fade away one by one!*

The tragedy is that although Seale Harris' work on hypoglycemia was published 25 years before Dr. Gyland became ill, none of the diagnostic specialists or prominent clinics were aware of it—or maybe they just refused to recognize it. Just imagine what that could mean to the patient with less persistence or skepticism than Dr. Gyland's regarding his own colleagues' infallibility? He could spend a fortune lying on a psychiatric couch treating his non-existent neurosis. Or, he could be operated on for a non-existent brain tumor!

The case of Miss A

Miss A is a beautiful actress, now very healthy, very successful, and very happy. Three years ago, she came to me in desperation. While on the verge of committing suicide, she was given by a friend and urged to read my newly published book, HOW TO GET WELL, which among other things, discusses the nutritional and biological treatment of hypoglycemia. After reading the section on hypoglycemia, she made an effort to contact me. Here is her story in her own words:

"After my second child was born, I became weak and apathetic, especially in the mornings. I couldn't get started until after two or three cups of strong coffee. Later in the day, I would get weak again, and extremely depressed. I was irritable all the time and gave a hard time both to my oldest child and to my husband. Sometimes, I would suddenly break out with a cold sweat. Some other times, I would break into tears for no apparent reason. At rehearsals, I couldn't concentrate on the script, my memory was bad, and the only way I could get through a performance was to drink a couple of cups of Irish coffee. Finally, at one performance, I not only forgot my lines, but I also fainted. I was told to quit working and see a doctor. My doctor gave me a complete physical checkup and, after taking over $200 worth of tests, he told me that there was nothing wrong with me physically; he referred me to a psychiatrist. This started me on three years of weekly visits to a psychiatrist. In the meantime, I started drinking more and more frequently, until I consumed two bottles of wine every day. My relations with my husband deteriorated more and more, until two years ago he left me completely. He took both children with him, since I was no longer able to take care of them. My psychiatrist finally suggested that I enter a mental hospital for 'observation and tests'; he also suggested that this may be the only way I could stop drinking. At the hospital, they diagnosed my condition as schizophrenia. I was given several drugs, I don't know what. Also, I was treated with electro-shock therapy. I was released from the hospital a year ago, but my health seemed to get worse since then. As soon as I stopped taking stimulant drugs, I could hardly move. I started drinking again huge amounts of coffee with lots of sugar. I was always exhausted, depressed, drowsy, and confused. I couldn't get work any more and I exhausted all my money on psychiatrists and doctors. Life became more and more unbearable. Finally, I couldn't see the point in living. Fortunately, I have many dear friends who stuck by me, and one of them brought me your book. That's why I'm here. You are my last hope. Please, can you help me?"

My first question, after she finished her sad story, was, "Have you ever taken a glucose tolerance test?" No, she didn't remember anyone giving her such a test. I said that before I would attempt to outline a therapeutic nutritional program for her, I would like to see such a test done. I referred her to a physician who I had been working with at the time. A few days later, she returned with the test results. The six-hour glucose tolerance test revealed not only an extremely low sugar level, but also an exceptionally fast drop. It was one of the worst charts I have seen.

The story has a very happy ending. After following the prescribed diet for three months, Miss A was not only able to gradually stop drinking coffee and alcohol, but her energy and vitality gradually returned, and for the first time in years, depressive and suicidal thoughts were replaced with increasing optimism and hope for a better future. The best part of all is that she is now again together with her husband and children and is hoping soon to resume her acting career.

Do you have hypoglycemia?

I will now list some of the long array of symptoms that are associated with hypoglycemia or caused by low blood sugar. Naturally, this will be a limited listing only, because to list *all* of the symptoms that millions of hypoglycemics experience would be to fill this entire book. As you read this list, I am sure you will find some symptoms that will apply to you. Does this mean that you have hypoglycemia? It may mean that—then, again, it may not. In the following chapter, I will show how, in addition to the patient's subjective description of symptoms, the doctor must use other diagnostic methods to arrive at a final and correct diagnosis.

Perhaps the most reliable list of the most common symptoms was given by Harry M. Salzer, M.D., psychiatrist, of the University of Cincinnati College of Medicine in Ohio. Dr. Salzer spent many years working with his own psychiatric patients, whose conditions proved to be caused by low blood sugar. Treating them nutritionally, he was able to restore their health and eliminate not only the somatic (physical) and neurological symptoms, but also the psychiatric ones. Dr. Salzer also points out that hypoglycemia can mimic any neuro-psychiatric disorders. Patients with low blood sugar have been diagnosed as having such illnesses as schizophrenia, manic-depressive psychosis, and psychopathic personalities.

Dr. Salzer became so interested in "problem hypoglycemia" that he later became the medical director of a foundation dedicated to research in hypoglycemia.[12]

Here is Dr. Salzer's list of the most common symptoms of low blood sugar, based on his questioning of over three hundred hypoglycemic patients whom he had treated. The symptoms are listed along with the percentages of patients complaining of them.[13]

Exhaustion	67%
Depression	60%
Insomnia	50%
Anxiety	50%
Irritability	45%
Headaches	45%
Vertigo	42%
Sweating	41%
Tremor (internal trembling)	38%
Tachycardia (palpitation of heart)	37%
Muscle pain and backache	33%
Anorexia (significant lack of appetite)	32%
Crying spells	32%
Phobias (unjustified fears)	31%
Difficulty in concentration	30%
Numbness	29%
Chronic indigestion	29%
Mental confusion	26%
Cold hands or feet	26%
Blurred vision	24%
Muscular twitching or cramps	23%
Joint pain	23%
Unsocial or anti-social behavior	22%
Restlessness	20%
Obesity	19%
Staggering	18%
Abdominal spasms	16%
Fainting or blackouts	14%
Convulsions	14%
Suicidal tendencies	10%

This is not all! Add to this the following symptoms which I have encountered in my work with hypoglycemics as well as those mentioned by Dr. Gyland on the basis of his experience in treating over six hundred hypoglycemics after he was cured from prolonged suffering of his own undiagnosed hypoglycemia:

Forgetfulness
Nervousness
Constant worrying
Ravenous hunger between meals
Indecisiveness
Lack of sex drive (females)
Craving for sweets
Impotence (males)
Moodiness
Allergies
Feeling of "going crazy"
Un-coordination
Itching and crawling sensations on skin
Gasping for breath
Smothering spells
Sighing and yawning
Unconsciousness
Night terrors, nightmares
Dry or burning mouth
Ringing in ears
Peculiar breath or perspiration odor
Temper tantrums
Hot flashes
Noise and light sensitivity

How many of these symptoms do you have? If you have a few, especially of short, passing duration, don't worry. Most people *at one time or the other* experience not just one, but many, if not most, of them. Remember, the key word is *passing.* Occasionally, we all may have most symptoms of hypoglycemia. If our sugar-regulating and emergency stress mechanisms work effectively, the body chemistry is quickly restored and health normalized—with symptoms fading away. But if you have an actual, untreated functional hypoglycemia, the symptoms may go away or change character, but they will soon reappear. You may have just a few of the listed symptoms, or you may have most of them, depending on the severity of the condition.

What should you do if you suspect having hypoglycemia?

My first advice is: Do not play doctor and do self-diagnosing. Go to a good nutritionally and biologically oriented doctor, who will, upon listening to your symptom description, suggest a six-hour glucose tolerance test. On the basis of the personal clinical examination (your subjective description of symptoms and how you feel), the results of the glucose tolerance test, and possibly a urinalysis and other tests if needed, your doctor will then be properly equipped to correctly diagnose your condition. If it is a clearly diagnosed functional hypoglycemia, ask him to treat you the way I suggest in this book—that is, if my therapeutic program for hypoglycemia makes common and scientific sense to you. And, if it doesn't, there is another, conventional, high-protein approach, which is also capable of alleviating the symptoms of hypoglycemia, although, as I will explain later, it does have harmful side effects. If you wish to consult a doctor who is familiar with my approach to the treatment of hypoglycemia, you may request a list of such doctors from the publishers—follow the procedure suggested at the end of the first chapter.

It is important that you follow the above mentioned diagnostic procedure. In the next chapter, I will describe the all-important Glucose Tolerance Test (GTT) and explain, both for the benefit of your doctor and yourself, how it must be read and interpreted. Fortunately, we have a steadily increasing number of enlightened doctors who understand the syndrome of hypoglycemia, so the chances that you will be mis-diagnosed are decreasing. Beware, however, of a doctor who, without tests, will dismiss your complaints with, "There is nothing wrong with you, it is all in your head."

Here are just a few of the mistaken diagnoses that thousands of hypoglycemics have received from incompetent doctors, or doctors who didn't "believe" in hypoglycemia and, consequently, didn't bother to test patients for it. The list is compiled from the reports by Drs. Gyland, Salzer, Fredericks, Martin, Weller, Cheraskin, and others.[2,7,10,13,14,15]

Mental retardation
Alcoholism
Neurosis
Diabetes
Menopause
Parkinson's syndrome
Rheumatoid arthritis
Chronic bronchial asthma
Allergy
Psycho-neuroticism
Cerebral arteriosclerosis
Meniere's syndrome (loss of hearing, dizziness associated
    with it, and noises in the ears)
Neurodermatitis (nervous skin disorders)
Chronic urticaria (hives)
Autonomic nervous system disorders
Brain tumor
Senility
Mental breakdown
Migraine
Epilepsy
Schizophrenia

This partial list of incorrectly diagnosed hypoglycemia shows how extremely important it is to have an absolutely correct diagnosis. Since hypoglycemia can mimic so many other conditions, the correct diagnosis can be extremely difficult and time-consuming. Because incompetent or over-worked doctors did not have time or interest to make an in-depth study and a thorough testing of their patients, thousands of hypoglycemics, whose conditions could have been cured by simple dietetic means, had their lives ruined, families destroyed, fortunes lost on psychiatric couches or mental hospitals, or were mis-diagnosed and treated with dangerous drugs and surgery for a long list of diseases they never had.

4

Glucose Tolerance Test

The standard and, at present, most reliable test for hypoglycemia is the glucose tolerance test, often referred to in medical terminology as the GTT. This test should be given in combination with a thorough clinical examination, history-taking, and carefully listening to a patient's own subjective description of the symptoms.

Unfortunately, some busy doctors do not have time to listen to the patient. I feel that it is extremely important to make a thorough survey of the patient's eating and living habits, and to listen carefully to his complaints. In professional seminars, which I periodically conduct for doctors, I recommend that those who practice nutritional and biological medicine allocate at least one hour, preferably two, for the initial consultation. Giving a glucose tolerance test without such thorough examination, could be not only useless, but even dangerous. Both doctors and patients must be aware that there are hypoglycemics who have no symptoms at all—on the other hand, there are patients with clear-cut symptoms of low blood sugar who have normal blood sugar levels. To make these obvious contradictions even more bizarre, there are people who show only minor abnormalities on the glucose tolerance test, but have severe symptoms of hypoglycemia; and some others with severe hypoglycemia who have comparitively mild symptoms. This is why I insist that an effective and safe diagnostic procedure includes all the means available to doctors, including a thorough exam and urinalysis, not just a five or six-hour glucose tolerance test.

There is another blunder that some doctors commit: giving a suspected hypoglycemic a three-hour glucose tolerance test. For diabetes a three-hour test may be sufficient. But, for hypoglycemia, a three-hour glucose tolerance test may completely miss the type of hypoglycemia that is actually most common—one which reveals itself only in the fourth, fifth, or even sixth hour of a six-hour test.[7,16]

How the test is performed

Perhaps, before we go into charts, I should explain to the lay readers how the six-hour glucose tolerance test is performed.

First, the patient is advised to go without food for several hours. If the test is given in the morning, as is most commonly done, the patient is advised not to eat anything after dinner the evening before, and definitely nothing after 10–11 P.M. Then, at the doctor's office, his first blood test is taken to determine the *fasting* blood sugar level. After that, he is given a glucose solution to drink. An hour after the glucose solution has been swallowed, another blood sample is taken. Five more samples are taken at hourly intervals and each is measured for its blood sugar level. Sometimes, in the first hour, also a ½-hour sample is taken.

In the *healthy* individual, the level of sugar will rise slightly, perhaps to 120, depending on where the fasting point was ("normal" span is considered to be between 80–120 mg. per 100 ml.); then, the sugar level will fall back to the normal range—to the fasting level before the test—or, for a short period, slightly below it, quickly returning to the normal.

In the *diabetic,* the level rises much higher than normal, perhaps to 200 or 300 mg., or even higher, and only very slowly goes down, not reaching the fasting level for six or more hours, depending on the severity of the condition. In *hypoglycemics,* however, the natural rise will be followed by a rapid drop below the normal fasting range. The *lower* and the *faster* it drops, the more severe the condition.

It is customary to take also a urine specimen each time blood is taken. The excess sugar is often excreted through the urine ("spilled" into the urine, as medical jargon calls it), especially in the case of diabetes. Because' hypoglycemia can often be confused with diabetes and because a patient may sometimes have both conditions intermittently, the urinalysis can be a valuable diagnostic adjunct to the blood test.

How to "read" tests

The fact that you were given a six-hour glucose tolerance test and that your doctor pronounced his verdict, is no guarantee that the diagnosis was correct. It all depends on your doctor's ability to "read the curve". There are so many variances in the curve of actual hypoglycemics, that unless your doctor has been specifically trained in this field, he may misinterpret the test results. This may happen, and does happen, so often because some doctors regard the certain, officially set blood sugar levels as "normal", and anything above or below that as "abnormal." For example, some official sources inform us that levels of blood sugar lower than 60 to 80 mg. are indicative of hypoglycemia.[17] The truth is that there are no set numbers or points which constitute hypoglycemia. Medical records show that some patients may experience severe reactions, both physical and/or emotional, although their blood sugar level never dips below 75 mg. Some people walk around symptom-free, while others demonstrate neurotic or even psychotic behavior on a virtually identical glucose tolerance test reading.

The most important factor to observe when attempting to read the glucose tolerance test chart is not *how low* the level drops, but *how rapid* the drop is. The drop from 200 to 100, when it happens in one hour or less, may cause more trouble in some persons susceptible to hypoglycemia than a slow, 2 or 3 hour drop from 100 to 50.

Also, the speed at which the glucose level *returns* to normal, and *how long it remains* at the low point, are extremely important factors to consider. The curve may drop pretty low, let's say to 50, but if it recovers quickly and returns to pre-fasting level, it may indicate a very mild case, often without noticeable symptoms. On the other hand, if the lowest point reads 65, but remains there for several hours, such a prolonged low level of blood sugar may result in very severe reactions.

In the following charts, I will try to show some of the typical, as well as not so typical, curve readings of patients with hypoglycemia. Also, for comparison, I will show the normal and the diabetic glucose tolerance test reading. In the text under each chart, the significance of the curve will be explained. Please understand that these graphic illustrations of the glucose tolerance tests are crude generalizations. In reality, *every patient* shows a different, individual curve, not more like anybody else's than his fingerprints are.

Please keep in mind that the GTT alone is *not* conclusive. It must always be used in combination with a clinical examination and a thorough history and symptom-taking.

Bill Gray, M.D. says, "Merely diagnosing hypoglycemia by abnormal glucose values is not enough. So-called 'normal' values are based on population averages and may not reflect what is normal for an individual patient. I ask patients to bring along a note pad and write down any symptoms that occur and the time they occur. To properly diagnose hypoglycemia, I insist on the complaints of the patients being correlated with the lowest point on GTT."[55]

NORMAL

Blood sugar curve range in healthy individuals (result of 6-hour test)

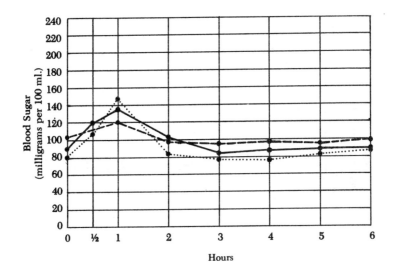

The three curves on the above chart are all within normal blood sugar levels. Note that although the rise is different, the drop is never, at any hour, too much below the starting point at fasting.

DIABETES

Diabetic range in mild and severe diabetes

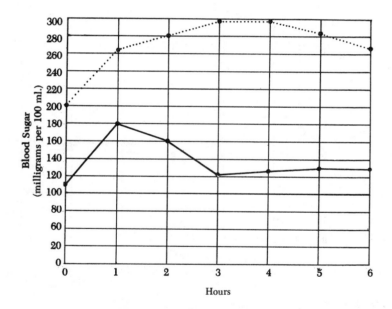

The solid line shows a mild diabetic blood sugar curve; the dotted line shows a severe diabetic curve.

HYPOGLYCEMIA I

Mild or pre-hypoglycemic curve

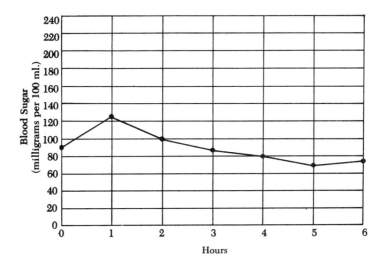

The above graph shows what Gyland calls a "pre-hypo-glycemic" curve. But even such a curve as this may result in many mild symptoms and, in some individuals, more severe symptoms. Also, according to a criterion devised by Dr. Herman Goodman, if the blood sugar one hour after break-fast—not after glucose dose—has not risen 50 percent or more above the fasting level, the patient is hypoglycemic. The above curve, then, is definitely suggesting hypo-glycemia, even though both readings fall within "normal range."

HYPOGLYCEMIA II
Mild

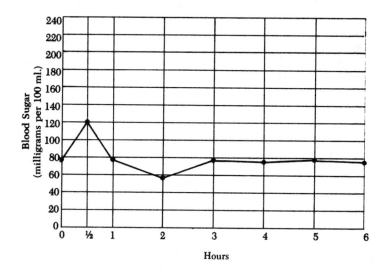

This is a mild form of hypoglycemia. Sugar drops to fasting level within the first hour and, after a further drop, goes up in the third hour to near fasting level. Although by the official "norms" this curve is supposed to represent *mild* hypoglycemia, the fact that the sugar drops rapidly 40 mg. in half an hour, may result in severe symptoms in some cases.

HYPOGLYCEMIA III

Common or classical forms

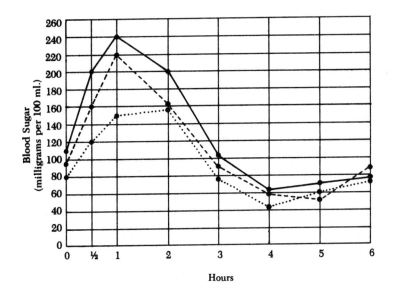

These three curves show a typical hypoglycemia curve: three hours after dose of glucose, the reading is lower than the fasting level. Notice also a rapid drop from a very high to a very low level.

HYPOGLYCEMIA IV

Normal beginning with severe hypoglycemic ending

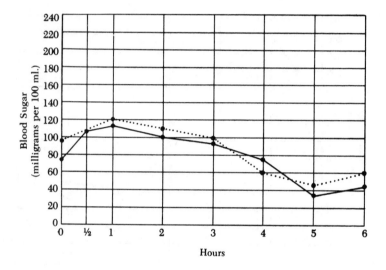

This curve shows a perfectly healthy response for the first three hours, but then the sugar suddenly drops and reaches an extreme low in the fourth or fifth hour. This is not uncommon at all and demonstrates the futility of trying to diagnose hypoglycemia by a three-hour glucose tolerance test.

HYPOGLYCEMIA V

Severe forms

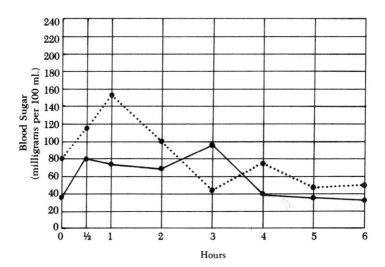

These two curves are typical of what are considered to be severe forms of hypoglycemia. The solid line shows sugar that is dangerously low at fasting time and never reaches any comfortable heights. The dotted line shows an almost 100 mg. drop within two hours which can result in severe hypoglycemic symptoms.

HYPOGLYCEMIA VI

Flat sugar-tolerance curve

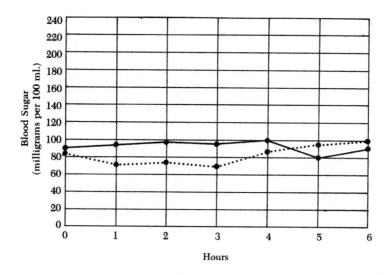

This graph shows the so-called "flat sugar-tolerance curve." Although some experts do not consider it to be true hypoglycemia, it is, in the author's opinion, a modified form of low blood sugar. Although the blood sugar does not drop to dangerous levels, it does not rise to normal comfortable levels either. This kind of curve sometimes appears in patients whose lives are monotonous, dull and unexciting. They complain of chronic fatigue, boredom, loss of zest and lack of libido.

Special important notes about GTT

Although the glucose tolerance test is at present an invaluable tool in diagnosing hypoglycemia, both doctors and patients should be aware of the following special considerations:

1. Patients undergoing a glucose tolerance test *must* tell their physicians (or be asked by physicians) if they have been taking the following drugs: cortisone, prednisone, or similar hormones; salicylates, such as aspirin, or other aspirin-containing drugs; diuretic drugs; oral contraceptives; or diphenylhydantoin (an anti-epileptic drug). The disregard of this caution may have severe repercussions and may even cause brain damage to the patient because of a violent reaction to the stress of the test itself on the drug-taking patient.

2. The GTT test in itself exerts a considerable *stress* on the person who is being tested. This stress may elicit the full-blown symptoms of low blood sugar in a patient who would otherwise react normally. This usually occurs at about the fourth hour of the glucose tolerance test. In some patients, psychotic behavior has been provoked by the stress of the test.

3. Because a six-hour GTT will take an obvious minimum of six hours, most such tests are conducted in the morning. It appears, however, that the body's own time cycles and biological rhythms intimately interact and/or influence the workings of the body's sugar-regulating mechanism. This is evidenced by the fact that some patients, whose reaction to the glucose challenge is abnormal in the morning, show a perfectly normal reaction if the test is given at noon or even later in the day.

Although some puzzled physicians who have observed this phenomenon could not decipher the cause of it, I think I can offer a fairly logical, as well as simple, explanation. Genetically and biologically programmed by millions of years of adaptation to environmental circumstances, one of which was that a heavy breakfast was never eaten early in the morning (food had to be obtained, caught, picked, harvested, etc., which took several hours), our body cannot handle the heavy insult of huge amounts of glucose (sugar) that is taken with tests given during the early morning hours. Since man traditionally consumed most food later in the morning, or at noon, the test given at a later hour would elicit a more natural response. Doctors may consider this when in doubt as to the significance of the GTT curve and possibly they could conduct an additional test at noon, or in the afternoon.

4. Bill Gray, M.D., a member of International Academy of Biological Medicine, and one of the leading biological medical practitioners in the country, whose report on his experience with the Airola Diet for Hypoglycemia appears in Chapter 11, has this to say about the glucose tolerance test:

"The best test would be values taken throughout the day during normal activity and normal diet. The problem with this is that there as yet is no standardization of such values. To be properly done, the glucose tolerance test should be done first thing in the morning after fasting since the previous evening. During the test, the patient should be encouraged to go out, take walks, be active. Sitting or lying around artificially raises the GTT curve, as discovered by tests done in hospitals."[55]

Causes of Hypoglycemia

In Chapter 2, I described the basic physiology and the mechanics of hypoglycemia and pointed out that faulty sugar metabolism is the main cause of functional hypoglycemia. Barring pathological conditions, such as pancreatic tumor, diseased liver, adrenal malfunction, or brain tumor—to name just a few of the most common medical problems that can be involved in hyperinsulinism, or low blood sugar—faulty eating and living habits are at the bottom of most cases of hypoglycemia.

Sugar

The primary dietary indiscretion that contributes to the development of hypoglycemia is a diet too high in refined starches (such as white flour and polished white rice) and refined white sugar. As stated earlier, Americans consume almost 125 pounds of sugar per capita per year. We also consume an equal amount of white flour in various forms. This is completely incredible nutritional folly; nothing less than an act of unintentional national suicide. An excess of sugar and refined carbohydrates in our diet is not only responsible for most of our hypoglycemia epidemic, but it is also a major contributing factor in an epidemic growth of most of our other degenerative diseases, such as diabetes, heart disease, tooth decay, periodontal disease, osteoporosis, and even cancer.[1,2,18] It is no wonder that white flour and white sugar are referred to by concerned scientists as the "white poisons" and the "white plague" of the civilized world. No lesser experts than John Yudkin, M.D., E. M. Abrahamson, M.D., E. Cheraskin, M.D., Weston Price, D.D.S., and J. I. Rodale—to name a few—have indicted excessive consumption of refined carbohydrates not only as the major cause of our physical degeneration, but also as a major contributing factor in the increased rate of crime and drug addiction, and in the epidemic deterioration of our mental and moral health. Far-fetched? See what Drs. Cheraskin and Ringsdorf, of Alabama University, say: "The sugar-laden American diet has led to a national epidemic of hypoglycemia, an ailment characterized by irrational behavior, emotional instability, distorted judgment, and nasty personality defects."[2] Much of today's irrational and anti-social behavior, on an individual as well as collective basis, can be traced to our denatured, chemicalized, nutritionless, sugar-laden diet. White flour and white sugar are more devastating to a person's health on an individual level, and to the physical, mental and social health of the whole human society, than any other single factor.[19]

There is a growing awareness among the general public today that "too much sugar is not good for you." Many housewives tell me "I don't use much sugar, and we only eat brown bread." How little they realize that almost everything that they buy at the supermarket today is loaded with sugar and/or white flour.

Soft drinks and ice cream are the worst of all, especially in view of the fact that they are consumed by children of all ages in astronomical quantities. Virtually all commercially produced bread, even so-called brown bread, not only contains added white flour, but also plenty of sugar. Candies, cookies, doughnuts, pies, cakes, frozen, canned, or prepared desserts, baby foods, dry breakfast cereals—all contain sugar, or white flour, or both. The only really effective way to eliminate these two health destroyers in our diet is to stop using any and all *man-made* foods and drinks, and to prepare your own food from scratch—from fresh vegetables, fruits, milks, cheese, nuts, grains, etc.—even begin to bake your own bread, which is not as difficult or bothersome as you may think (see Chapter 13 for instructions). Speaking of making food from scratch, the following story illustrates how far we have departed from our traditional, inherited right, responsibility, and ability to prepare our own food. Fed-up with eating warmed-up canned soup every day, the newlywed husband finally protested to his bride, "Honey, why don't you try to make soup from scratch, like my mother used to do?" Offended, but determined to please her husband, the wife was busy at the supermarket the following day searching all over for the ingredients for a home-cooked soup. Finally, she called the manager and complained "I am looking all over, but I can't find it—where do you keep scratch?"

Why sugar is "bad"

White sugar and white flour are not whole, natural foods. They are refined, fragmented, adulterated and denatured. Sugar cane and sugar beet are whole natural foods. White sugar made from them has been completely stripped of all nutrition present in the original food. All minerals, all vitamins, all trace elements, enzymes, fatty acids, and amino acids (proteins) have been removed in the process of refining the sugar. The final result is a pure crystallized form of sucrose, a white, pharmaceutically pure chemical.

Everything I said about white sugar applies more or less to white flour. Although the whole grain is rich in complex nutrition, in the process of refining flour, practically all the vital nutrients have been destroyed or removed, leaving a nutritionless white powder, which is mostly a pure starch. If that is not bad enough, in order to destroy the last traces of life and make it snow white, the processors treat the flour with toxic chemical bleaches and conditioners.

Eating white sugar and white flour presents three problems:

1. Eating such denatured, devitalized, demineralized, and devitaminized foods will inevitably lead to nutritional deficiencies.

2. Since our bodies are genetically and physiologically equipped to effectively metabolize *only* natural whole foods, (the genetic ability being determined by millions of years of use and adaptation) eating fragmented, refined foods, from which essential synergistic and complexed elements have been removed, will lead to metabolic disorders and biochemical imbalances. For example: white sugar is not only an empty-calory food, stripped from all the vitamins and minerals, but in order to digest and process (metabolize) it, the body must use its own supplies of minerals and vitamins, which may lead to both deficiencies and imbalances in the body's own stores of vital nutrients.

3. Since our bodies are not equipped to process refined, concentrated foods, continuous ingestion of them will exert a great strain on many organs and glands. The continuous strain and abuse of these organs can damage them and cause their paralysis and malfunction.

This will bring us to hypoglycemia which is, more than by any other factor, caused by malfunctioning glandular and metabolic systems, especially by the malfunction of such organs as the pancreas, the liver, the adrenals, and other endocrine glands. And, the excess of refined carbohydrates in the diet, especially of white sugar and white flour in all forms, as well as the excess of other concentrated forms of carbohydrates, such as alcoholic beverages, sweetened juices, and soft drinks, is the prime contributing factor to the continuous stress on these vital organs and glands which leads to their malfunction and breakdown.

How sugar contributes to hypoglycemia

Whole, complex, carbohydrate foods, such as whole grains, fruits, and vegetables, are digested slowly and changed into forms of sugar that the body can use for energy and for its various vital functions (in Chapter 2 we described this process in detail). But refined starches and concentrated refined sugar are quickly absorbed into the bloodstream, thus raising the blood sugar to dangerous levels. This triggers an emergency action on the part of the insulin-producing pancreas. The normal variations in the blood sugar levels, which occur when meals of natural, whole foods are eaten, do not trigger any abnormal reactions from the pancreas. But when refined, concentrated sugar is consumed and the blood sugar level rises quickly, the "panicked" pancreas over-reacts and dumps an excessive amount of insulin into the bloodstream to counteract the dangerously high sugar level. The excessive insulin not only brings the sugar level down, but does two things that are responsible for a long list of unpleasant symptoms and personality changes:

- It lowers the sugar far *below* normal (normal being the fasting level in each individual).

- Drops the sugar level *too fast.*

Too low, too fast!

When sugar drops too low, and especially if it does it rapidly, several of the body functions are severely impaired. Heart and muscle action are weakened. Brain and nerve activity are deranged. Energy and endurance level are lowered. Emotional stability and control are lost. This is why the hypoglycemic in this state craves a quick pick-up, preferably sweets, coffee, caffeine-containing soft-drinks, alcohol, or certain drugs, which rapidly remedies the unpleasant symptoms by bringing the blood sugar level up. Since these artificial stimulants with their swift, drug-life effect, raise the sugar level too high, the pancreas is again forced to over-react and counteract the dangerous situation by over-producing insulin. This creates the typical vicious cycle of the hypoglycemic: hyperactive, happy, and energetic for a short time when the sugar level is high; and totally exhausted, confused, and ready to jump out the window a few hours later.

Coffee

The studies demonstrate that coffee raises the blood sugar level in diabetes, but drastically lowers the blood sugar level in victims of hypoglycemia. This is not as contradictory as it may seem. Sugar does the same: it raises the sugar level in diabetes and lowers it in hypoglycemia because of the hypoglycemic's over-reacting pancreas. Dr. E. M. Abrahamson tells of patients whose hypoglycemia was controlled by proper diet, but who had violent blood sugar reactions when they took as little as one cup of coffee.[19] Coffee has a stimulating effect on the adrenal glands which, in turn, encourages the liver to release more sugar into the blood.

The combination of coffee and sugar is particularly harmful. Sugar enters the bloodstream quickly and directly, while coffee adds to the total sugar level by acting through the adrenals, brain, and liver.

Considering how popular coffee is in America and how much of it is consumed daily, coffee very well may be one of the major contributing factors to our hypoglycemia epidemic.

Caffeine-containing beverages and drugs

Cola drinks are even worse than coffee. In addition to a high caffeine content, they are loaded with an incredible amount of sugar, plus dangerous phosphoric acid—a perfect combination to keep your dentist busy!

You may not be aware that, besides coffee and cola drinks, some commonly used over-the-counter drugs can add considerably to your total daily ingestion of caffeine.[20] Look at this list:

Brewed coffee, cup	100–150 mg. caffeine
Tea, cup	60–75 mg. caffeine
Cola drinks, glass	40–60 caffeine
Aspirin, Bromo-Seltzer, tablet	32 mg. caffeine
Excedrin, tablet	60 mg. caffeine

Excessive caffeine ingestion, either from coffee, or caffeine-containing beverages and drugs, produces a long line of typical hypoglycemic symptoms: anxiety, light-headedness, heart palpitations, nervousness, agitation, irritability, trembling hands and muscle twitches, and insomnia. All symptoms usually disappear as soon as the patient stops drinking coffee or caffeine-containing beverages.

Alcohol

Most experts agree that there is such a condition as alcohol-induced hypoglycemia. Dr. John W. Tintera, who made an extensive study of the alcohol-hypoglycemia link, says that the crux of the alcoholic problem can be traced to low blood sugar.[8] Dr. Robert Atkins says: "Experience shows that when an alcoholic succeeds in getting off alcohol, he usually substitutes sweets. This is because almost all alcoholics are hypoglycemic, and sugar provides the same temporary lift that alcohol once did."[21]

For a non-alcoholic, an occasional drinker, a night of heavy drinking may produce low blood sugar the "morning after", with all the classic symptoms of hypoglycemia. In fact, the symptoms of a hang-over are nothing but symptoms of hypoglycemia. But for the alcoholic, low blood sugar can become a chronic condition. According to Dr. S. J. Roberts, alcohol reduces the output of glucose by the liver, which may precipitate or exaggerate low blood sugar.[28]

The relationship is reciprocal. Chronic drinking, just like excessive sugar in the diet, contributes to the development of hypoglycemia; and, a person with hypoglycemia is a potential candidate for alcoholism. When he finds that alcohol produces the same effect as sugar, he becomes a compulsive drinker. A dangerous viscious cycle ensues: alcohol improves his sense of well-being only temporarily, so it becomes necessary for him to drink most of the time in order to feel comfortable and symptom-free. He has become a chronic drinker, an alcoholic.

Tobacco

It has been shown in actual human studies that smoking causes a rapid blood sugar rise with just as rapid a drop in blood sugar level shortly after the cigarette or cigar is put out. A Swedish study, reported in a prestigious British medical journal, Lancet, showed that in some study subjects, the rise of blood sugar was as high as 36 percent. Nicotine in tobacco was isolated as the culprit, since a comparable test with denicotinized cigarettes did not produce the same effect as regular cigarettes. The Swedish researcher concluded: "The rapid fall of the blood sugar level after the smoking throws further light on the habit of chain smoking—the craving for another pick-me-up . . ."[22]

An American study by M. G. Barr, M.D., showed that a group of heavy smokers who all suffered from typical symptoms of hypoglycemia—emotional instability, apprehension, insecurity—and whose glucose tolerance tests showed similar curves to those of functional hypoglycemics, did not respond to the low blood sugar diet. Only a total halt of smoking led to the disappearance of symptoms as well as to a normalization of blood sugar levels.

Of course, the reader must be aware that hypoglycemia is not the only—or even the worst—problem that can be caused by smoking. The relationship of smoking and cancer is well-known and well documented.[23]

Smoking also can cause severe vitamin C deficiency. There is a disagreement among various investigators as to *how* this deficiency is caused. Dr. W. J. McCormick, one of the most knowledgeable men on the subject and the world's leading authority on vitamin C (with whom I had the great privilege of studying the vitamin C subject in the mid-50's) claimed that nicotine "destroyed" vitamin C at an approximate rate of 25 mg. per cigarette.[24] Some other researchers speculate that vitamin C is not actually destroyed, but is used in the process of detoxification of toxic products of smoking—vitamin C being an acknowledged detoxifier. However, according to more recent Canadian studies, conducted with the assistance of the Canadian government by Dr. Omer Pelletier, smoking apparently interferes with the body's ability to *utilize* vitamin C.[25]

Whatever the actual mechanism of the tobacco-caused vitamin C deficiency, the lesson is the same: Smoking is a severe health hazard, especially for hypoglycemics or potential hypoglycemics. Vitamin C deficiency is linked to disorders in the sugar control mechanisms.

Salt

Excessive salt intake also contributes to hypoglycemia by causing a loss of blood potassium which leads to a drop in blood sugar. Potassium is necessary to rectify sugar metabolism abnormalities. Again, as is almost always the case with hypoglycemia, the reverse relationship can be established even in regard to salt. Excessive salt intake causes potassium losses, which results in a drop in the blood sugar level—the low blood sugar level triggers the onset of stress, causing much potassium to be lost in the urine and causing sodium, as well as water, to be retained in the system (this is known as edema or water retention). The administration of potassium chloride in such cases quickly raises the blood sugar level and eliminates the unpleasant symptoms of hypoglycemia.[26] Sometimes, potassium tablets can be useful for hypoglycemics, especially those who are prone to blackouts.

The inordinate desire for salt experienced by some hypoglycemics, can be a symptom of possible adrenal failure. Malfunctioning adrenals, by permitting abnormal salt excretion, encourage heavy salt consumption. And, as I mentioned earlier, the inefficiency or malfunctioning of the adrenal glands is almost always causatively involved with the development of hypoglycemia. The adrenal glands do need some salt for normal functioning; therefore, total abstinence from salt is not advisable. The hypoglycemic should use a moderate amount of salt, but only from natural sources such as whole sea salt, kelp, or sea water.

Food allergies

It has been known for a long time that hypoglycemia may initiate or aggravate allergies. Now, it also is clear that allergies may cause hypoglycemia. Persons who suffer from food allergies can, after an initial rise, experience a significant drop in blood sugar level when exposed to allergens—as much as from normal levels all the way down to 30. This is low enough to cause severe symptoms.[27]

The causative relationship between food allergies and hypoglycemia is not difficult to understand. The allergic person's body regards allergens (substances to which it is allergic) to be poisons, and treats them accordingly by making an heroic effort to neutralize, excrete, destroy, or combat them. Thus, allergens cause a severe stress on the system. And *all* stress, especially on a continuous basis, may contribute to low blood sugar, mostly by straining the adrenal glands and causing adrenal exhaustion.

Allergies other than those to food, such as allergies to automobile exhaust, pesticides, dust, any of the household chemicals and detergents, food additives, and even such "small" things as vapors from a marking pen, or specific brands of cosmetics or perfume, can trigger the body's defensive mechanisms, and cause the consequent drop in blood sugar level.

Emotional stress

Emotional stress can cause hypoglycemia as any stress can. And, certainly, hypoglycemia can be a cause of much emotional stress. One type of hypoglycemia in particular is linked causatively with emotional stress. It is a kind that is characterized by a "flat glucose-tolerance curve" (see Chapter 4 for a chart that graphically illustrates that curve).

Flat-curve hypoglycemia is a type of low blood sugar that is not dramatic or extreme, but it nevertheless has a devastating effect on a person's life and his functions as a human being. It is caused by what Dr. Sydney A. Portis calls "pernicious inertia."[33] This is a disturbance in sugar metabolism that is usually found in patients whose life is as flat as their test curve: uninteresting, without zest, without challenge. Often, they are forced into occupations or life situations that offer no excitement or challenge. They react with "apathy, loss of zest, a general let-down feeling of aimlessness, a revulsion against the routine of everyday life, be it occupational activity or household duties", as eloquently defined by Dr. Portis. When a person finds no challenge and no sense of accomplishment in pursuing his unpleasant and unescapable duties, his body responds to the deficit in mental and emotional challenge with equal apathy and inertia: there is poor, discoordinated, weak action of the two organs that deal with mental and physical challenges, the adrenals (which elevate blood sugar) and the pancreas (which lowers it). The result is a chronic low-grade cerebral starvation. As another psychiatrist put it, "A condition of emotional letdown, based upon the disruption of the patient's goal structure, influences the vegetative balance and manifests itself in a disturbance of the regulatory mechanisms controlling the sugar concentration of the blood."[34]

The flat-curve hypoglycemic is usually feeling "half alive", complaining of constant fatigue, existing in a twilight zone where apathy, exhaustion, disinterest, lack of motivation and boredom are typical symptoms. His sugar levels do not dip low enough to cause blackouts or other dramatic symptoms, nor do they rise high enough to permit efficient functioning or to bring some zest into his life.

Our American way of life creates plenty of prospective candidates for flat-curve hypoglycemia: the housewife, stuck with monotonous, unrewarding, tedious, repetitive duties; the business executive who sees no prospects of promotion and has resigned himself to performing his duties routinely; the car washer, the cashier, the bookkeeper, the assemblyline worker—all performing dull, repetitive chores without a sense of achievement; all living the lives of what Thoreau described as "quiet desperation." No wonder physicians find more and more cases of this undramatic form of hypoglycemia. And the only reason they do not encounter it even more is because the condition is not severe or dramatic enough to warrant a worried call to a doctor—people just continue enduring their uneventful, dull, boring, and zestless lives.

I dwelled extensively on this specific type of hypoglycemia because

1. It is only seldom correctly diagnosed. In part, because the person suffering from it does not recognize that he is sick; and, in part, because physicians are not sufficiently trained to read the GTT charts and often miss the existence of the condition.

2. If left untreated, flat-curve hypoglycemia may develop either into full-fledged hypoglycemia or into diabetes.

3. This condition can be remedied by a combination of dietary therapy with psychological counseling that can motivate the patient to a change of life-style and life-orientation.

Nutritional deficiencies

Since the major cause of hypoglycemia is the derangement, malfunction, or breakdown of sugar metabolism regulating mechanisms, consisting largely of the pancreas, the liver, the adrenals, thyroid, and pituitary gland, it stands to reason that anything that can contribute to the damage of these glands and organs can be looked upon as causative factors in hypoglycemia. Nutritional deficiencies can either cause or aggravate almost any ailment, and hypoglycemia is no exception.

There are several specific nutrients that are involved in sugar metabolism. Deficiencies (or sometimes excesses) of these nutrients can disrupt the normal metabolic processes or contribute to the breakdown or malfunction of organs involved with sugar metabolism. I will mention some of these:

Chromium. Chromium is one of the trace elements needed for proper sugar metabolism in the body. It has been shown by a growing amount of research that the lack of chromium can cause the impairment of the blood sugar regulating machinery which is controlled by insulin. According to Dr. Walter Mertz, a physician-nutritionist of the U.S. Agricultural Research Service, chromium is required by the body to manufacture the Glucose Tolerance Factor (GTF), which regulates blood sugar. When an individual is not getting enough chromium, he suffers from impaired glucose tolerance. This is of specific importance in diabetes, but chromium deficiency can also have an unfavorable effect on the victims of low blood sugar.

It is also well known that there is a severe chromium deficiency in the American diet. Dr. Doisy of State University of New York Upstate Medical School Center in Syracuse, has been testing especially elderly Americans for their chromium content. He found that they have much less chromium in their bodies than people of a like age in the Middle or Far East, and in more primitive nations in Africa. And Dr. Kenneth M. Hambridge, of the University of Colorado Medical Center, by using hair analysis, found that Americans of all ages are suffering from chromium deficiency.[29]

Brewer's yeast is one of the best supplements for the hypoglycemic. In addition to supplying a wealth of nutrients, as you will see from the next chapter, it is one of the few excellent food sources of chromium. In addition, brewer's yeast also contains the Glucose Tolerance Factor, which seems to make the chromium more available to the body. Dr. Doisy has found that by giving yeast to patients who had disorders in glucose tolerance, he was able to stabilize their blood sugar levels within a month. He also found that brewer's yeast could prevent attacks of low blood sugar.

Zinc. Zinc is closely tied to the body's use of insulin. Zinc is plentiful in the healthy pancreas, where insulin is manufactured, and, actually, is a constituent of the hormone, insulin. It appears that zinc is lacking in people who suffer from low blood sugar and/or diabetes. Zinc is also essential for all healing.

The best natural sources of zinc are whole grains, seeds, and nuts. Most zinc is removed in the processing of white flour. Zinc is now also available in tablet form and is sold in all health food stores. The daily supplementary dose should be between 10 and 30 mg.

Vitamins B and C. Both of these vitamins increase the body's tolerance to sugars and carbohydrates and help to normalize sugar metabolism. The deficiency of these vitamins is widespread in the United States, especially the deficiency of B vitamins which are removed or destroyed in the processing and refining of grains. Brewer's yeast is an excellent source of all B-complex vitamins.

Pantothenic acid. The deficiency of pantothenic acid has been specifically singled out by extensive research as a major contributing factor both in hypoglycemia and in adrenal exhaustion. It has been found in studies with diabetics that if pantothenic acid is undersupplied in the diet, the blood sugar drops so quickly after insulin is given that the danger of insulin shock, or a blackout, is tremendously increased.[30,31] This is of extreme importance to the hypoglycemic since *the rapidity* of the drop of sugar is the most dangerous aspect of the hypoglycemic glucose-tolerance curve. It is not how low, but how fast, sugar drops that is significant. The body can tolerate reasonably well a gradual drop in sugar level, but cannot quickly adjust to a sudden drop. When the brain and other vital organs and muscles are suddenly left without sufficient glucose and the oxygen it carries, they react with most unpleasant symptoms.

If a deficiency in pantothenic acid can contribute to or accelerate the rapid drop in blood sugar level, it would seem that the hypoglycemic should make sure that he never allows a risk of undersupplying his body with this important nutrient.

Brewer's yeast is, again, an excellent source of natural

pantothenic acid. The other good sources are wheat germ, wheat bran, whole grain breads and cereals, beans, peas, nuts, liver, egg yolk, green vegetables, and royal jelly. Of course, to make sure that this all-important vitamin is always supplied in abundance, hypoglycemics or those who are predisposed to hypoglycemia and wish to avoid it, should take supplementary pantothenic acid in tablet form. It is available in all health food stores. The usual dosage is 100–200 mg. per day. (See Chapter 9 for the recommended supplements for hypoglycemia.)

Magnesium, potassium, vitamin E, and vitamin B6 are other nutritive substances the deficiency of which has been linked with hypoglycemia.[9,50]

In addition to the above mentioned nutritional factors that are connected with the development of hypoglycemia, there is another very important factor which has been totally overlooked by virtually all researchers. This factor is—now brace yourself for a shock!—the overconsumption of protein, especially meat. This is paradoxical, indeed, since a high-protein diet with an abundance of meat is the very diet usually recommended by orthodox doctors and nutritionists as a treatment for hypoglycemia!

Let's look at this perplexing question in the next chapter.

The Folly of the
High-Protein Diet

The standard hypoglycemia diet recommended by most orthodox practitioners and nutritionists in the United States is a high-protein, low-carbohydrate diet, the so-called Seale Harris diet, named after Dr. Harris who first described the disease and who also devised a diet to treat it. This was in 1924.

Over fifty years have passed, but the standard hypoglycemia diet is still the same. Fifty years ago, nutrition research was in its early infancy. Most vitamins had not yet been discovered. The understanding of biochemistry and metabology was limited. Nutrition generally was not considered to be related to disease, except in such conditions as diabetes, pellagra or kwashiorkor. Furthermore, protein was considered to be *the* most important food element, a nutritional panacea. When Dr. Harris devised his high-protein diet for hypoglycemia, he had no idea that such a diet, which would supply excessive amounts of protein, would be anything but beneficial to the general health of the patient. He found in his clinical experience that a protein-based diet was able to control the symptoms of low blood sugar. He had never suspected that the huge amount of protein that hypoglycemics would consume on a daily basis in following his diet, could possibly be harmful to the patient in some other ways. The orthodox thinking on protein at that time was "the more the better!"

Fifty-five years later, and especially during the last decade, the scientific consensus regarding protein and its relation to health and disease, have undergone dramatic changes. From all over the world, scientific research is turning out new evidence almost daily which shows that:

- our views on protein were erroneous and are in need of a thorough overhaul;

- our daily need for protein is much less than was previously believed; and,

- an *excess* of protein in the diet can be extremely harmful and may contribute to the development of many degenerative diseases, including our worst killers, heart disease and cancer.

And, as far as hypoglycemia is concerned, while it is true that a high-protein, low-carbohydrate diet will control symptoms in severe hypoglycemics, it actually will aggravate the condition in the long-run and make it incurable. It has been well established by reliable studies that a high-protein, low-carbohydrate diet is extremely taxing on the adrenal glands, overstressing them and causing them to break down. Even the advocates of the high-protein diet admit that such a diet is certainly no cure, and it offers no real recovery, since it must be maintained indefinitely.

In addition to heart disease[35] and cancer, especially cancer of the colon[36,37], current studies indicate that excessive protein, especially excessive meat consumption, is dangerous in many other ways. It may contribute to the development of such serious degenerative conditions as kidney damage, osteoporosis[39], atherosclerosis[35,38], pyorrhea[39], arthritis[40], and even senility and premature aging[41].

Now isn't it the height of folly to advise a treatment that merely replaces one illness with a host of others? Does it really make any common or academic sense to you when a doctor tries to control a non-fatal condition with a therapy that may cause other, more serious, or even fatal diseases?

But then, this has been our orthodox, drug-oriented, symptom-focused medical approach for some time. Doctors treat symptoms with drugs, which instantaneously wipe out the symptoms. No one seems to be concerned with the fact that the "recovered" patient will be back soon with perhaps even more severe problems caused by the "miracle drugs" he took a few days or weeks earlier. Then, a set of new drugs will take care of his new symptoms, and so on. . . . A vicious cycle, a dreadful failure on the part of our medical establishment to see the patient as a whole, physical, emotional, and spiritual complex entity, and to try to *cure a sick individual*, not just to treat the *symptoms* of his ill health.

The orthodox treatment for hypoglycemia with a high-protein, low-or-no-carbohydrate diet could be rightfully referred to as a case of the "remedy being worse than the disease." If doctors would adhere to the first principle of the art of healing and live up to the essential part of the Hippocratic oath they took—"Primum est nil nocere" (the most important is that treatment does no harm)—they would think twice before advocating such a dubious therapy. The fact that our medical establishment has failed to come up with a safer diet for hypoglycemia than the outdated Seale Harris diet, even when it is evident that this diet is potentially dangerous, is a grave indictment against the establishment doctors for their inability to keep abreast with scientific research. Instead of directing their efforts toward removing or controlling the symptoms, they should have devised a therapy that would take into consideration the patient's total health and welfare.

Facts, fads, and fallacies about protein

Americans have been subjected for several decades to never-ending high-protein propaganda. This brainwashing, sponsored by livestock, dairy, and meat industries, has succeeded in convincing us that we need "lots and lots" of protein for good health. The result is that Americans today eat more protein than people of any other nation in the world. Our average protein intake is between 100 and 110 grams daily. However, instead of enjoying better health, as anticipated, we have progressively more disease than does the rest of the world. Our life expectancy is in 21st place among the nations, we are 18th in terms of infant mortality, and we lead the world as far as cancer, heart disease, osteoporosis, diabetes, and hypoglycemia is concerned.

The scientific fact that our bodies are built largely of proteins may have contributed to the high-protein cult. Proteins are very important nutrients and we need lots of them every day for the various functions within the body. They are needed for: the repair and rebuilding of cells; the synthesis of enzymes and hormones; mineral metabolism, etc. But how much is "lots"?

Our leading nutrition experts have been advocating 120, 150, or even more grams of protein a day. In fact, we have been made to believe that the more protein we consume, the better. We just couldn't get too much of it! Yet, the most recent world-wide research shows that the actual daily need of protein in human nutrition is far below that which has long been considered necessary. Finnish studies by Dr. V. O. Sivén; American studies by Drs. R. Chittenden, D. M. Hegstead, and W. C. Rose; Swedish studies by Dr. Ragnar Berg; Japanese studies by Dr. Kuratzune; and finally German studies by Prof. K. Eimer—all show that protein intake between 25–35 grams a day is sufficient to sustain good health.[42] And recently, Dr. Ralph Nelson, of the Mayo Clinic, confirmed older studies by Dr. Eimer and Dr. Chittenden, which show that the performance of athletes improved on a lower protein intake.[43]

Perhaps the following fact will convince you more than anything else. The Food and Nutrition Board of the National Academy of Science, in collaboration with the World Health

Organization, publishes every four years the Table of Recommended Daily Allowances of various nutrients. In the last two decades, they have lowered the daily recommendation for protein from 120 grams to only 46 grams! Why? This was prompted by world-wide scientific consensus and the growing concern that an excess of protein in the diet, just like an excess of anything else, can be extremely harmful and can contribute to the development of biochemical and metabolic imbalances and diseases.

Let us now examine some of the other commonly held myths about protein.

Animal versus vegetable protein

Proteins are made up of 22 amino acids, which are the building blocks of protein. Most of these amino acids are synthesized within your body, but 8 amino acids are not, and therefore must be present in foods you eat. They are called the *essential* amino acids. Those foods that contain all eight essential amino acids are called "complete protein foods"; those that are missing one or more of the essential amino acids are called "incomplete protein foods."

According to outdated and erroneous thinking, only animal foods, such as meat, fowl, fish, milk, and eggs, contain complete high quality proteins, but proteins in vegetable foods are inferior or incomplete. The newest nutrition research has now completely disproved the validity of such thinking. Studies made at the most respected nutrition research center in the world, the Max Planck Institute in Germany, show that the earlier beliefs about the biological superiority of animal proteins were unsubstantiated, and that many vegetable protein foods are "just as good or better than animal proteins." Vegetable foods which contain all eight essential amino acids, and, therefore, are complete protein foods, are soybeans, peanuts, almonds, buckwheat, sunflower seeds, pumpkin seeds, potatoes, avocados, and all green leafy vegetables.[44]

In addition, even those vegetable foods that do not contain all the essential amino acids and which, consequently, are not complete protein foods, will become useful and biologically complete protein foods when properly combined with each other. For example, corn and most beans are incomplete protein foods, each being low in some essential amino acids. Luckily, amino acids missing in corn are ample in beans; and, amino acids missing in beans are well-represented in corn. Thus, the combination of tortillas and beans, a famous dietary staple of Central, South and some parts of North America, is an excellent source of high-quality, complete proteins.

Excess protein spells ill health

Here are some other important facts about protein:

1. Overconsumption of protein, especially of meat, can cause severe deficiencies of vitamins B_6 and B_3 because both of these vitamins are needed in abundance to metabolize proteins. Since they are largely missing in meat, they are drawn from the body's own stores.[45]

2. One of the dangerous by-products of animal protein metabolism is ammonia. Ammonia has been recently found to be a strong carcinogen and one of the causes of cancer of the colon.[36]

3. Excess meat in the diet can cause a severe calcium and magnesium deficiency. The reason: meat contains 22 times more phosphorus than calcium. Since these two minerals are needed in about equal amounts in the diet, this excess of phosphorus will cause depletion of the body's own calcium stores, since phosphorus cannot be properly digested without extra calcium. The result: osteoporosis, osteoarthritis, pyorrhea and periodontal disease, tooth decay, and other calcium deficiency related diseases.

4. Too much protein in the diet can contribute to the development of mental disorders, particularly schizo-

phrenia, as reported by famed Russian researcher, Dr. Yuri Nikolajev.

5. Too much animal protein in the diet can lead to premature senility by causing a biochemical imbalance in body tissues, overacidity, intestinal putrefaction, constipation, and degeneration of vital organs.

I wish to stress two other important discoveries about proteins that were reported by the Max Planck Institute:

1. Vegetable proteins are not only equal to, but they are actually *superior* in biological value to those of animal sources. For example, the proteins in potatoes are biologically superior to the proteins in meat, eggs, and milk. And just think—in common American thinking, potatoes are berated and looked upon as a pure starch food.

2. Raw proteins have a higher biological value than cooked proteins. Cooking makes all proteins less assimilable. You need only about one-half the amount of proteins if you eat raw vegetable proteins instead of animal proteins, which are, as a rule, cooked.[46]

I have good reason for this long discussion of the issue of protein. Since my hypoglycemia diet, which will be described in the next chapter, is based on a low-animal-protein, high-natural-carbohydrate principle, I wanted you to fully comprehend the reason for my departure from the conventional hypoglycemia diet, which is a high-protein, low-carbohydrate diet. I believe that any therapeutic diet should not only be corrective or useful in the treatment of the condition for which it is prescribed, but should also comply with the following two principles that cannot be compromised:

• It must do no harm to the patient.

• It must be beneficial for the general health of the

patient—it must improve, rather than endanger his total health.

As you have seen in this chapter, the high-protein diet cannot meet the above-mentioned requirements. Although it will admittedly help to control the symptoms of hypoglycemia, it can be extremely harmful to the patient if used for any extended period of time. My diet, on the other hand, will not only control the condition, but it will actually help to correct it permanently by normalizing the functions of pancreas, adrenals, and other vital organs and glands, and by contributing to the betterment of the total health and well-being of the patient.

The above discussion of the protein issue must not be construed as an attempt to de-emphasize the importance of protein. Proteins are, of course, vital nutritive factors and certainly necessary in any diet, including the diet of the hypoglycemic. But because something is good doesn't mean more is better! It is *not protein*, but *too much protein* which is "bad." We are so brainwashed by two decades of protein-oriented propaganda that although we readily accept the fact that too much fat is harmful (although fat is vital in human nutrition), that too much carbohydrate is harmful (although carbohydrates certainly are important), and that too much of *anything* is not good, we have an almost allergic resistance to the mere suggestion that too much protein, also, can be undesireable!

7

Airola Diet
for Hypoglycemia

If you are not now experiencing the symptoms of low blood sugar but, on the basis of the reading of the preceding chapters of this book, are motivated to do everything you can to prevent the development of hypoglycemia, you can do it by following the dietary, supplementary and other special programs and exercises that are recommended in this and the following chapters.

By and large, the Airola Diet for optimum health should also be followed by those who suffer from hypoglycemia, with some exceptions mentioned in the text.

So, here it is:

The optimal nutritional program for prevention and treatment of hypoglycemia

PROHIBITED FOODS

The following foods and drinks should be completely excluded from your diet:

1. White sugar and everything made with it. This means: ice cream, pastries, cookies, candies, breakfast cereals, soft drinks, commercially baked breads, etc.

2.   Even other forms of sugar, such as brown, raw, turbinado, and fruit sugar, should be avoided. Honey can be used, but only in strict moderation—not more than ½ tsp. at a time, maximum 1 teaspoon a day.

3.   White flour and everything made with it: bread (much of commercially sold bread, although it is labeled as brown or whole-grain bread, contains white flour), packaged breakfast cereals, cookies, pastries, pies, gravies, etc.

4.   All soft drinks, root beers, and so-called juice-drinks. Even those drinks that are sugar free, must be avoided. Remember: it is not only the sugar and the refined carbohydrates that contribute to the development of hypoglycemia, but anything that damages your health generally and causes extra strain and stress on the system. Artificial sweeteners and artificial flavorings, as well as phosphoric, citric, and other strong acids added to even sugar-free soft drinks, are definitely harmful and should be avoided.

5.   Coffee and caffeine-containing soft drinks, such as colas.

6.   Alcohol and tobacco.

7.   Excessive amounts of sweet fruit or vegetable juices, even if they are natural and without added sugar. Example: carrot juice, grape juice, apple juice, orange juice—all contain large amounts of sugar which can be harmful for hypoglycemics, especially those who are super-sensitive to concentrated carbohydrates; they even can contribute to the development of hypoglycemia or diabetes in those who are healthy.

8. All processed, canned, refined, and other denatured supermarket-sold, man-made foods, even TV dinners and breakfast cereals. Buy only fresh foods, grains, vegetables, fruits, milk, etc., and prepare your own meals.

9. An excess of protein, especially meat. An adequate nutrition, including all the required proteins, can be obtained from the diet suggested in this chapter. If you insist on eating animal protein foods, a moderate amount of meat or fish can be allowed, perhaps once a week, but their addition to the diet is not necessary.

THE OPTIMUM DIET

Your basic diet should be made up of these three food groups (in this order of importance):

A. Grains, seeds, and nuts.
B. Vegetables.
C. Fruits.

A. **Grains, seeds, and nuts** are the most important and potent health-building foods of all. Their nutritional value is unsurpassed by any other food. Eaten mostly raw and sprouted, but also cooked, they contain all the important nutrients essential for human growth, sustenance of health, and prevention of disease in the most perfect combination and balance. In addition, they contain the secret of life itself, the *germ,* the reproductive power that assures the perpetuation of the species. This reproductive power, the spark of life in all seeds, is of extreme importance for the life, health and reproductive ability of human beings.

All seeds and grains are beneficial, but you should eat predominantly those that are grown in your own environment. Sprouting increases the nutritional value of seeds and grains; hypoglycemics should eat as many sprouts as possible. Wheat, mung beans, alfalfa seeds, and soybeans make excellent sprouts.

As we mentioned in previous chapters, soybeans, buckwheat, sesame seeds, pumpkin seeds, almonds, and peanuts all contain *complete proteins* of the highest biological value. But the protein in all seeds and grains, even those that do not contain *all* the essential amino acids, is extremely useful if the foods are combined and eaten together.

Seeds, grains, and nuts are not only excellent sources of proteins, but also the best natural sources of essential *unsaturated fatty acids* without which health cannot be maintained. They are also nature's best source of *lecithin,* a substance which is of extreme importance to the health of the brain, nerves, glands (especially sex glands), and arteries.

The *vitamin* content of grains, seeds, and nuts is unsurpassed, especially vitamin E and B-complex vitamins. Vitamin E is extremely important for the preservation of health and prevention of premature aging. And B-complex vitamins are absolutely essential for practically all body functions, but they are particularly needed by the hypoglycemic because they are very much involved in protecting the body against stress. They are directly involved in sugar metabolism and the sugar control mechanisms. Vitamin B deficiency can also damage the adrenal cortex, which is often at the root of low blood sugar problems.

Grains, seeds, and nuts are also gold mines of *minerals and trace elements.* It is becoming more and more apparent that minerals are even more important to health than the more glamorized vitamins. A balanced body chemistry, especially in terms of acidity and alkalinity, is dependent on minerals. Biochemical disorder in the system, of which sugar metabolism disorder is one manifestation, is a basic underlying cause of most disease. Grains and seeds are the best sources of such trace elements and important minerals as magnesium, manganese, iron, zinc, copper, molybdenum, selenium, chromium, flourine, silicon, potassium and phosphorus. Sesame seeds are an excellent source of calcium. Molybdenum, which is still a very much ignored mineral, is present in many whole grains, especially in brown rice, millet, and buckwheat, and is involved with proper carbohydrate metabolism. Magnesium, zinc, potassium, chromium, and manganese are also of specific importance to hypoglycemics because they are involved in normalizing sugar metabolism.

Grains, seeds, and nuts also contain *pacifarins,* an antibiotic resistance factor that increases man's natural resistance to disease. They also contain *auxones,* natural substances that help produce vitamins in the body and play a part in the rejuvenation of cells, preventing premature aging.

The importance of whole grains and seeds in the diet has been recently emphasized, stressing their bulk and roughage content. After several decades of eating refined and processed foods, from which the outer coating, the bulk, has been processed out, man has become plagued by constipation, diverticulitis, colitis, and cancer of the colon and intestinal tract. The current studies show that to avoid this epidemic, we must go back to whole, unprocessed grains and seeds, which provide enough bulk to prevent these disorders.

The best seeds for the hypoglycemic are: flax seeds, sesame seeds, chia seeds, and pumpkin seeds. Sesame seeds are an excellent source of easily digestible and assimilable calcium. Tahini and other sesame butters can also be used. They are sold in health food stores.

Flax seeds are an excellent food, largely neglected in the American diet. The extraordinary nutritional value of flax seeds is based on the fact that they contain a great amount of the highest quality essential fatty acids, such as linoleic and linolenic acids, or vitamin F factors. Flax seeds are also a highly mucilaginous food and are very beneficial for the healthy workings of the alimentary canal and eliminative system. They are an excellent food to prevent and/or remedy constipation. Keep in mind, however, that flax seeds and sesame seeds contain 45–50 percent fat; so do not overeat—they can be fattening.

The best nuts are: almonds, peanuts, hazelnuts. Almonds are, in terms of rancidity, the most durable of all nuts, even when they are shelled. They also supply complete, high quality proteins, as sesame and flax seeds do.

All seeds and nuts must be eaten *fresh* and *raw*. Nuts can be chewed (but well!) and seeds should be ground in your own seed grinder (available at your health food store for about $12) just before eating. Remember, ground flax seeds will turn rancid within a few hours, so it is better to grind them fresh and eat them at once.

I did not mention another popular seed food, sunflower seeds, because it is increasingly more difficult to get sunflower seeds that are not rancid. They are extremely vulnerable to rancidity and turn rancid quickly after they are shelled. How will you know if your seeds are rancid? Spread them on a white paper and notice all the seeds that are not medium grey, but are, in whole or in part, brown, yellow, white, black—these are all rancid. Even a small quantity of rancid seeds can be extremely toxic and harmful, even carcinogenic, if consumed often.

Nuts and seeds are of specific importance to hypoglycemics. As you will see from the suggested menu in the next chapter, hypoglycemics should eat several small snacks between meals. Raw nuts, especially almonds, are excellent for this purpose. They can be carried in your pocket or handbag and eaten when a pick-up is needed.

Nuts and seeds combine beautifully with fresh fruit for breakfast, a most suitable breakfast food for hypoglycemics.

The best grains for hypoglycemics are buckwheat and millet, although most grains are useful and beneficial. Since wheat is one of the most common allergens (foods that cause allergy in many people), and since allergy is so often involved in hypoglycemia, those suffering from low blood sugar must be sure they are not allergic to wheat before they incorporate it as a part of the diet. If eating wheat in any form (even wheat germ) gives you any trouble, such as gas, indigestion, stomach pain, and increased pulse rate, leave it out completely.

Millet is the best cereal for hypoglycemics (see Chapter 13 for the best ways to prepare millet). Millet contains an unusual carbohydrate that does not adversely affect hypoglycemics. It is very easily digested and supplies an adequate amount of good proteins, minerals, and other nutrients.

Buckwheat is another excellent cereal. According to the U.S. Department of Agriculture, the proteins in buckwheat are complete and are of such high biological value that they are comparable to proteins in meat. Buckwheat is also an excellent source of magnesium and manganese, both extremely vital for hypoglycemics. Zinc is also well supplied by buckwheat.

Important question: cooked or raw?

If you have read even a minimal amount of health and nutrition literature, you must be aware that most experts highly recommend eating as many foods as possible in their natural, raw state. I am no exception. Cooking destroys some of the nutritive value of food. Proteins and fats are damaged by heat and become less assimilable. Some of the vitamins, especially C and B, and a considerable amount of minerals can be leached out if the food is boiled in water for a long period of time. Steam cooking, crock-pot-cooking, or waterless cooking is definitely preferable. The frying of food, especially if it is done in vegetable oils, can be hazardous, since vegetable fats become carcinogenic if heated to extremely high temperatures, as in frying. (Frying in animal fats is safer since they are more resistant to damage by extreme heat.) Cooking also destroys all the enzymes in foods, as well as any other life-factors that are present. Any way you look at it, the general rule of healthful eating seems to be that as many foods as possible, perhaps up to 80 percent of the total calory intake, should be eaten in their natural raw state.

But there are some important exceptions to this rule, as there are to any rule. Fanaticism in nutrition can be dangerous. Unfortunately, some uncompromising fanatics who are "into" raw foods, refuse to recognize that in the science of nutrition (which is, like medicine, not an exact science, but rather an art), there are always exceptions, compromises, and special considerations. This is only natural since there is a great physiological, biochemical, and structural difference between different individuals, and because our present nutrition has evolved through thousands of years of search, selection, and environmental adaptation. An example: Man has been eating a great variety of initially wild, then cultivated plants (vegetables). Many of these plants are excellent and edible in their raw state. But some plants contain too many harmful substances, such as oxalic acid, for example, and man, therefore, avoided them. However, with the discovery of fire, man has learned to use even these plants, by destroying or leaching out the harmful elements through cooking. Thus, spinach, rhubarb, asparagus, cauliflower, cabbage, and other vegetables of the cabbage family, have become part of a regular diet. In a raw state, especially if consumed in large quantities, they can be quite harmful.

The story of beans is somewhat similar. Many beans, especially soybeans, contain enzymes that inhibit the body's protein utilization. Man discovered very early that eating beans raw led to digestive disorders, mineral and protein deficiencies, and other discomforts: He has found that these foods became more useful if cooked. Cooking destroys the enzyme-inhibitors and makes digestion and assimilation of these foods better. Thus, cooked soybeans became an essential part of man's diet in the Orient. But soybeans can also be eaten raw if they are first soaked for 24 hours in water which is changed every 6 hours. The enzyme-inhibitors are thus soaked and leached out from the beans.

There is another important factor—the most important in fact—that must be taken into consideration when dealing with the question of cooked or raw foods. Minerals in all dry grains and most dry beans, peas, and other legumes, are chemically bound with phytic acid, or phytin. If grains or beans are eaten very fresh, like raw corn on the cob, or raw soft peas or beans, they can be digested fairly well and the mineral content in them can be sufficiently utilized. But dry grains or beans, if eaten raw, or if just soaked overnight, cannot be digested properly and the minerals in them will be largely wasted and excreted with the phytins to which they are chemically bound. Cooking grains, as in baking bread or making porridge or cereals, helps to break down this chemical bond and releases all the vital minerals such as zinc, iron, manganese, magnesium, molybdenum, etc., making them easily available and assimilable in the intestinal tract.

To avoid misunderstanding and confusion, let me summarize. All seeds and nuts, and all fruits and most vegetables, should be preferably eaten in their natural state— raw. Some vegetables, like those mentioned above, should be cooked, preferably boiled in water, discarding the water. But all grains should be either cooked, like in bread or cereals, or sprouted. Sprouting also breaks down the phytin and releases the minerals.

Now, if at this point you are oriented toward 100 percent raw food eating, you may conclude, "Great, even if I am convinced of the importance of eating grains, I still don't have to cook them—I'll just sprout them!" This is an excellent solution if you insist on a nothing but 100 percent raw food diet—BUT, it is still not the right approach if you are suffering from hypoglycemia. Most hypoglycemics must eat at least some of their grains cooked. Here is the reason.

Raw grains, like wheat sprouts or sprouted beans, digest relatively fast, as do most raw foods, in comparison to cooked foods. However, quick digestion and utilization of carbohydrates from grains is *not* what we want in the hypoglycemia diet. It is imperative for the maintenance of even, sustained sugar levels in the blood that the assimilation of carbohydrates be as slow as possible. And cooked cereals, such as buckwheat or millet, or whole grain breads, digest much more slowly than raw cereals, releasing sugar into the bloodstream gradually and at a slower pace. This is extremely important in the preventive as well as therapeutic diet for hypoglycemia. When you eat a bowl of buckwheat cereal, oatmeal, a five-grain cereal, or millet cereal, for lunch or breakfast, along with a dab of butter, or a tablespoon of vegetable oil, and a glass of fresh raw milk, such a meal will remain in your stomach for many hours—half a day!—slowly releasing high quality proteins, fatty acids, and gradually converted starches (sugars) into your bloodstream.

This same principle also indicts the animal proteins as a bad choice for hypoglycemics. Animal proteins are digested relatively rapidly. Only the protein needed by the body at the time of digestion is utilized as protein. The rest is changed into sugar and burned as energy food, or is deposited as fat. A very moderate amount of animal protein in the hypoglycemia diet would not present serious problems, but if a patient eats a typical, conventional high-protein diet, the above mentioned factor and its ramifications should be considered.

B. **Vegetables** are the next most important food group in the Optimum Hypoglycemia Diet. Vegetables are extraordinary sources of minerals, enzymes and vitamins. Most green, leafy vegetables contain complete proteins of the highest quality. The proteins in alfalfa, parsley, and potatoes are comparable to the protein in milk in their biological value.

Most vegetables should be eaten raw in the form of green salad. In fact, one meal of the-day, lunch or dinner, should be largely made of vegetables (see Menu in the next chapter). Some vegetables, such as potatoes, yams, squashes, green beans and those mentioned earlier as containing an excess of toxic acids can be cooked, steamed, or baked.

Garlic and onions are excellent health-promoting as well as medicinal foods and should form an important part of the hypoglycemia diet. Garlic and onions contain special sugar-regulating factors. Garlic and onions, complemented by a large assortment of natural herbs and spices, will help to improve your health as well as turn dull vegetable dishes into delectable gourmet foods.

There is a vegetable (actually, botanically, it is a fruit, but dietetically it is mostly used as a vegetable) that is of extraordinary value in the hypoglycemia diet—avocado. Avocado contains a special kind of sugar, a 7-carbon sugar, known as mannoheptulose, which does not stimulate insulin production, and, in fact, *actually suppresses it.* This makes avocado an excellent choice of food for hypoglycemics, and possibly an unwise one for some diabetics. Mannoheptulose, this special insulin inhibitor, is present in many natural foods, but avocado seems to be one of its best sources.[47]

Hypoglycemics should take advantage of this especially useful food and eat it as often as they can. While most other concentrated foods will have the effect of raising the blood sugar, avocado will actually do the opposite. Avocado also happens to be a food that contains complete nutrition: that is, it contains protein, fats, carbohydrates, minerals, and vitamins in excellent proportions. It does, however, contain over

16 percent fat, so those who have tendencies to overweight should not eat huge amounts of avocado—maybe one small, or one-half of a larger avocado a day.

Other vegetables that are specifically beneficial for hypoglycemia as well as for diabetes are string beans and Jerusalem artichokes. Artichokes can be eaten raw, in salads. String beans are best steamed. Both vegetables contain *inulin* which is converted into levulose in the body. Levulose is a form of fruit sugar that is well tolerated by the body without unfavorably affecting blood sugar levels.

C. **Fruits** are listed in the third, and last, place in importance in the Optimum Diet for hypoglycemics. This is because most fruits contain large amounts of easily available sugars which can cause a rapid blood sugar rise if consumed in quantity. Fruit juices, especially, must be consumed in strict moderation.

Hypoglycemics should choose fruits that are not excessively sweet, such as sour apples, cherries, strawberries, papaya, grapefruit, lemon, lime, and pineapple. Dried fruits should be largely avoided, unless soaked in plenty of water or, possibly, used as a part of cooked cereals. Grapes, grape juice, and dates should be avoided by those whose condition is severe, but they are allowed in very small amounts in the diet of those whose cases are mild.

The best way to eat fruit is in the raw state, *in season,* and preferably in the morning, for breakfast. One-half banana, one apple, a slice of fresh pineapple, ½ cup of fresh berries, ½ grapefruit—these are good choices, especially if combined with a handful of fresh, raw nuts and/or seeds of your choice. One glass of kefir, yogurt, or other forms of soured milk can be eaten with this meal.

Fruit is also a useful snack food between meals.

Just keep in mind this most important fact about fruit or fresh fruit juice: you don't have to eliminate them from your diet if you eat and drink only *small* quantities at a time. You may even eat dates if you wish—but only *one* date at a time! All sweet fruit juices should be diluted 50–50 with water, and not more than 1 or 2 oz. consumed at any one time.

Lemon is one fruit that is of specific importance for hypoglycemics. Lemon is an excellent stimulant and rebuilder of the liver. The liver function is involved in keeping a proper sugar balance. A tired, overworked, or toxic and malfunctioning liver is almost always causatively involved in sugar metabolism disorders. A 3-day liver detoxifying treatment, as described on page 122 in HOW TO GET WELL[6], when a glass of lemon water is drunk every two hours, is a splendid way to rejuvenate a congested, toxic or malfunctioning liver. (Fresh red beet juice, 1 oz. at a time, is another effective way to help the rebuilding of the liver and the improving of its functions.)

SUPPLEMENTARY FOODS

A diet comprised of foods from the above mentioned three basic food groups will provide you with all the nutritive factors needed for maintenance of optimum health, prevention of disease, and long life. This diet can be supplemented with other excellent foods, if desired. This supplementation is especially recommended for "beginners", those who are now eating the regular American diet of sugar, white bread, meat, and canned junk foods and who wish to switch to more healthful eating habits. With these added supplementary foods, it will be easier to prepare meals and make sure that an adequate amount of all the essential nutrients is provided by the diet.

Milk and milk products

Although the value of milk in human nutrition has been highly disputed in some American nutrition circles, most nutritionists in Europe and leading nutritionists in this country agree that milk can be an excellent, even indispensible, addition to the human diet.

In the hypoglycemia diet, milk and milk products can play an especially important role, particularly when meat is not eaten. Milk protein can be a valuable addition to the total vegetable protein supply. Milk is also an excellent source of valuable minerals, particularly calcium.

The fatty acids of milk are well balanced and supply saturated and unsaturated fat—both forms being important in human metabolism. In this age of the cholesterol scare, we have been brainwashed to think that saturated fats and cholesterol, which are present in meat or butter, are nothing but villains, causing cholesterol deposits in the arteries as well as numerous other undesirable effects. The truth is that dietary cholesterol has only a very insignificant effect on the amount of cholesterol in arteries. The excessive use of refined carbohydrates, such as white sugar and white flour, is the biggest villain in this regard, contributing indirectly to pathological cholesterol levels in the body.[18] As far as saturated fats are concerned, we now understand that our body needs both saturated and unsaturated fats. Milk and butter provide both, and if used along with vegetable oils in the diet, will provide a pretty balanced supply of the fatty acids needed for all vital body functions.

The best way to consume milk is in its soured form: yogurt, kefir, acidophilus milk, piima;, madzoon, buttermilk, or plain clobbered milk. I am constantly asked, "Which of these is best?" The answer is: all fermented, soured milks have approximately the same nutritive and health-building value, which is mainly due to their lactic acid content and to their exceptional digestibility, as well as to their beneficial effects on intestinal flora and the health of the digestive and eliminative tract. Soured milks are superior to fresh milk because they are, in fact, *predigested* foods and are, therefore, very easily assimilated. So, when choosing your soured milk, feel free to be guided by your own taste preference—they are all beneficial.

Natural, cultured cheeses are also excellent foods for hypoglycemics, as is cottage cheese, especially homemade kvark (see Chapter 13). Cheese slices or chunks can be easily carried to work or on travels, can be used as snacks and pickups when needed between meals, and can possibly be interchanged with nuts and fruit, or even eaten along with them. A glass of kefir or buttermilk goes well with a fresh fruit meal, or with a vegetable meal. With a cooked cereal meal, fresh milk is preferable.

Needless to say, when I recommend supplementing the diet with milk and milk products, I mean only the *highest quality, uncontaminated, raw, unpasteurized milk from healthy animals.* High quality milk and milk products are often sold in health food stores. Today's pasteurized, supermarket-sold milk is loaded with toxic and dangerous drugs, hormones, chemicals, residues of pesticides, herbicides and detergents. Such milk is not suitable for human consumption. I can only recommend natural, raw, "farmer's" milk. Note that Scandinavians, Bulgarians, Russians—the people we always associate with remarkable health—are traditionally heavy milk users, but they use it mostly in soured forms.

For hypoglycemics, soured milks are of a special importance. In soured milks, the milk sugar, or lactose, has been changed into beneficial lactic acid. So, while sweet milk contains some sugar, which, in extreme hypoglycemics, can trigger hyperinsulinism, sour milk is largely free from sugar and is safe to eat.

After making all these glowing and favorable remarks about milk, I must issue a warning. Many people are either allergic or intolerant to milk!

Milk is one of the most common allergens. Since some hypoglycemics suffer also from allergies, you must make sure that you are not allergic to milk before you incorporate it into your therapeutic hypoglycemia diet. If you feel discomfort after eating milk or cheese, if you get stomach pains, gas or diarrhea, you may suspect an allergy. In such a case, you should leave milk and milk products completely out of your diet at least until your health is normalized, your resistance to stress is increased, and your allergic reaction to milk is eliminated.

Now, about milk tolerance. There are a great number of people who are milk intolerant. They cannot properly digest milk or cheese, which give them nothing but gas and digestive problems. Why? Dr. Robert D. McCracken, anthropologist at the University of California School of Public Health, explained this simply and logically. The descendants of the countries wherein the inhabitants historically herded dairy animals and traditionally lived on a lactose-rich diet (milk, cheese, etc.), are usually tolerant to milk. Their intestines contain the enzyme, *lactase*, which breaks down milk sugar, *lactose*, into a form that the body can use. Thus, milk for them is an excellent health food. Conversely, those whose ancestors never or seldom used milk as a major element in the diet, are usually intolerant to milk because their intestines do not contain sufficient lactase.

So, if your ancestors come from Europe, Scandinavia, or the Middle East, it is likely that your body is genetically programmed to use milk and digest it effectively. If your ancestors are from Africa (except the East African Nilotic Negroes), China, the Phillipines, or other areas where milk was not traditionally used, it is likely that your body is not programmed to digest milk properly.*)

As a final comment regarding milk, it should be pointed out that goat's milk is better than cow's milk as a human food. Its mineral and protein composition is closer to human milk, and its fat is easily digestible because it is naturally homogenized. Goat's milk is also usually free from contaminants.

---

*) By the way, you *cannot* change this genetic programming in just a few generations—it would take thousands of years to accomplish this.

Cold-pressed vegetable oils

High-quality, fresh, cold-pressed, crude, unrefined, unheated, and unprocessed vegetable oil is recommended in moderate quantity as a regular addition to the diet. Please reread the foregoing sentence and notice all the specifications and requirements that I place on vegetable oil before I can recommend it for human consumption. Such oils are almost impossible to obtain today.

All commercially produced, supermarket-sold oils are a complete no-no. They are all produced either with the use of extremely high temperatures, up to 350°F, or with the process known as chemical extraction, in which such solvents as hexane and benzine are used. Both methods result in a final product which has no resemblance to anything "natural." It is processed, refined, bleached, and deodorized. Lecithin, which normally clouds the natural unrefined oils, has been removed. Toxic chemical antioxidants, such as BHT, have been added. Margarines, made from such vegetable oils, have, in addition, been saturated with hydrogen and are even worse than the original oils they are made from.

But even most oils sold in health food stores are not actually cold-pressed. Some manufacturers use a misleading term, "cold-processed", which really means that the oils were extracted with the help of chemical solvents, such as carcinogenic hexane. There are only a very few oils that can be made by hydraulic pressure, and, thus, can be truthfully labeled as cold-pressed. Sesame seed oil and olive oil are among these few oils. For example, there is no such thing as cold-pressed wheat germ oil, even if the label states that. Most oils are extracted by a screw-type press. This method results in extremely high temperatures. The oils are heated to 300–350°F. There is evidence that exposing vegetable oils to such high temperatures makes them carcinogenic.

In addition to these hazardous manufacturing and processing methods, there is another danger connected with edible oils. All natural foods are extremely perishible, and vegetable oils are no exception. Natural oils turn rancid very fast. It is almost impossible to keep them for any length of time without the use of preservatives. Keeping in metal cans or dark bottles helps. Also, constant refrigeration is essential. Even then, most oils will turn rancid within a few weeks or months after they are made. Wheat germ oil is almost always rancid.

Here is a riddle: Vitamin E is a natural antioxidant. According to some experts, adding vitamin E to oils will prevent their oxidation and rancidity (rancidity is caused by oxidation). Why, then, does wheat germ oil, which contains more vitamin E than any other oil, turn rancid extremely fast, while sesame seed oil, which has a very low vitamin E content, is one of the most durable oils existent in terms of rancidity? Indeed, the longer one studies nutrition, the more mysteries one encounters!

So now what? Should we leave all oils completely from the diet? How can we get truly safe edible oils?

Since my book, ARE YOU CONFUSED?, which pioneered the information on the danger of eating rancid foods and oils, was published a few years ago, many changes have taken place in the American health-oriented segment of the edible oil industries. An effort is now being made to produce better oils. I cannot mention brands or manufacturers' names in my writings, but there are now several brands of better quality natural oils available. Ask for these oils in your health food store. If your store does not have them, they will get them for you. Some stores sell a good imported brands of virgin olive oil from France, Italy of Spain.

The best edible oils are olive oil and sesame seed oil. These are also the two oils most likely to be non-rancid.

Olive oil is of special interest in the hypoglycemic diet since it is an excellent source of the important fatty acid, arachidonic acid, which is needed for the synthesis of prostaglandins within the body. Prostaglandins are involved in balancing hormonal levels and may be of importance to proper sugar metabolism which is controlled by hormones.

Warning: *Never use vegetable oils for cooking or frying;* use them only in their cold state on salads and on cereals or other dishes, approximately one tablespoon a day. If you need some fat for occasional frying or sauteeing, use butter. Never use oil in baking bread. Use my bread-making recipe which does not require oil (see Chapter 13).

Honey

Natural, raw, unrefined, unfiltered and unheated honey is the only sweetener allowed in the hypoglycemia diet, but only in strict moderation: 1 tsp. a day, ½ tsp. at a time, for sweetening of herb teas, or for use on food. This allowance is largely for children and older people. Honey possesses many medicinal properties; among others, it is beneficial in kidney and liver disorders and in problems with poor circulation. If used sparingly, it will not have a significant blood sugar elevation effect. However, in extreme cases of low blood sugar, even honey must be completely excluded from the diet.

Brewer's yeast

Here is a special supplementary food that is extremely useful in the hypoglycemic diet. It is beneficial both for the prevention and the treatment of hypoglycemia.

The value of brewer's yeast as an indispensible supplement in the hypoglycemic diet is based on the following properties:

- Brewer's yeast is an excellent source of high quality proteins. When meat is left out of the diet, brewer's yeast can complement the vegetable sources of protein in the diet.

- Brewer's yeast is the best food source of B-vitamins. B-complex vitamins are essential for proper carbohydrate digestion and utilization. B-vitamins are also needed to keep vital organs and glands working properly. They particularly support the activity of the adrenal glands and the liver—the organs directly involved in sugar metabolism.

- Brewer's yeast is the best anti-stress food known to man. It is also a rich source of specific anti-stress vitamins: B_1, B_6, B_{12}, and pantothenic acid.

- Brewer's yeast is an unmatched source of the trace minerals which are specifically involved in sugar metabolism and provide healing factors in hypoglycemia: selenium, iron, zinc, and chromium. Yeast contains the Glucose Tolerance Factor which is vital to sugar regulation and tolerance.[48] This is of great importance both for hypoglycemics and for diabetics. Selenium is similar to vitamin E in many of its functions. Since some hypoglycemics seem to be unable to tolerate large doses of vitamin E (over 200–400 IU a day) selenium supplementation in the form of brewer's yeast can be of value to them. Zinc, as a constituent of insulin, is also involved in carbohydrate and energy metabolism.

The best way to take brewer's yeast is to use it as a snack food. As you will see in the following chapter, the most prominent feature of the hypoglycemic diet is snacking—eating several small snacks between the main three meals. One tablespoon of brewer's yeast powder mixed in a half glass of freshly made or canned pineapple juice, or freshly squeezed grapefruit juice, can be taken 2–3 times a day, preferably one hour before meals. Taking brewer's yeast in this manner will also totally eliminate an explosive problem too often associated with the consumption of yeast—gas. Brewer's yeast should never be taken *with meals,* or immediately before or *after* meals, as is generally the case with other vitamin and mineral supplements. Yeast contains up to 50 percent pure protein. Protein needs lots of hydrochloric acid to be effectively digested. To assure trouble- and gas-free digestion, brewer's yeast should always be taken on an empty stomach, when there is a plentiful supply of hydrochloric acid.

There are many food yeasts on the market. When I mention yeast in my lectures, I am always beseiged by questions: Which of the numerous available yeasts is the best? Although all food yeasts or primary yeasts are useful in human nutrition, for hypoglycemics the true *brewer's yeast* is best. By "true" I mean the real yeast that is a by-product of the brewing industry. Not "brewer's-type" yeast, not "primary" yeast, not "torula" yeast, not just a "number so and so" yeast, but one which is labeled "brewer's yeast." True brewer's yeast is a better source of selenium and chromium, and of the Glucose Tolerance Factor, than any other form of yeast. In all fairness, I must say that the all-important B-vitamins are present in approximately the same quantities in all food yeasts.

Special important notes on yeast:

1. When taking yeast, always take one tablet of calcium supplement with it. Yeast is rich in phosphorus and low in calcium. An addition of calcium will achieve a better mineral balance and improve the utilization and metabolism of all of the yeast's minerals. As a calcium supplement, bone meal, calcium lactate, dolomite, or calcium-magnesium tablets can be used; or you can take calcium-rich sesame seeds. Even taking the yeast with some form of calcium-rich soured milks, such as yogurt, kefir, acidophilus milk (buttermilk), etc., can be helpful.

2.   Never eat *live* yeast intended for baking. Live yeast may multiply in the intestines and, instead of supplying you with B-vitamins, may actually consume your body's own B-vitamin reserves.

HEALTH-PROMOTING EATING HABITS

Not only what you eat, but *how you eat* is very important. The cliché you often hear, "You are what you eat", is a flagrant example of oversimplification that is frequently used in the field of nutrition. The phrase "You are not what you eat, but what you assimilate" would be much closer to the truth.

The effective assimilation and utilization of nutrients from the foods you eat is dependent on many factors. Let's look at some of them.

1. Eat only when hungry.

There are all kinds of theories regarding eating and drinking—when you should or should not eat or drink—theories invented by scientists. They tell you that you should eat a large, heavy-protein breakfast, with meat, liver, eggs, etc., first thing in the morning, whether or not you are hungry that early in the morning. They tell you when to eat heavy meals and when to eat lightly. They also tell you when and how much to drink. Much such advice is based on unsubstantiated, pseudo-scientific notions. You don't need any scientists or their theories to tell you when and how much to eat. *Nature* has provided a built-in mechanism within your brain which will tell you unmistakeably *when* you should eat or drink. You should eat when you are hungry and drink when you are thirsty. Contrarily, you should *not* eat when you are *not* hungry, nor drink when you are *not* thirsty. This is the best possible guidance upon which you can rely. Your requirements for food and drink are unique, different from everybody else's. But you never go wrong if you closely follow your hunger and thirst signals.

Food eaten without appetite will do you no good. It will, in fact, harm you by overburdening the digestive organs with unwanted materials and creating indigestion, gas, and other disturbances. For the hypoglycemic, this means extra, unnecessary stress on the body and extra dietary sugar at a time when the body doesn't need it.

2. Eat slowly in a relaxed, unhurried atmosphere.

Slow eating and thorough mastication are essential for good digestion. Good chewing is especially advisable for hypoglycemics, since carbohydrates are partially digested in the mouth with the help of digestive enzymes present in the saliva, and they are even partially assimilated directly through the membranes of the mouth. This will help to stretch out the time during which all carbohydrates are assimilated, which is an asset for hypoglycemics.

Good chewing and slow eating make you feel satisfied sooner and with a smaller amount of food. This is important in view of the fact that many hypoglycemics have a weight problem and often are obese. Food should be "Fletcherized", chewed throughly at least 40 times for every mouthful.

Also, food should be eaten in a relaxed atmosphere and *enjoyed.* Biologically, only the foods eaten with genuine pleasure will do you any good. A peaceful, unhurried, and happy atmosphere around the table will pay good dividends in improved digestion and assimilation of food—and, hence, in better health.

3. Eat several small meals during the day in preference to a few large meals.

This is especially important to hypoglycemics, and to those who wish to prevent the development of both diabetes and hypoglycemia. But anyone would benefit from adhering to this rule. In fact, judging from my observation and studies of various peoples and their eating habits, I can hypothesize that the fact that so many Americans eat only two or even one large meal a day, may be responsible in part for our high prevalence of hypoglycemia. I have found that in more "primitive" countries known for their excellent health, people always eat several small meals a day. In addition to two or three main meals, they have some snacks in between as they go about their usual work. Watching people work in the fields in Russia and Ukraina, I noticed that they interrupt their work every two hours or so to eat and/or drink a little something: a fruit, a glass of sour milk, a watermelon, a plate of cold summer borsch, or whole fresh vegetables, such as cucumber, tomato, or carrot—or just a slice of black sour bread with onions. Come to think of it, this is a perfect diet for hypoglycemics or for the prevention of low blood sugar! When a Mexican laborer goes to work, he takes with him several oranges, mangos, ever-present limes, or a large jicama, and he has a snack of something every now and then. No wonder hypoglycemia is unheard of in Russia or Mexico.

Snacking can also lead to reducing. It has been shown in actual studies that while 1500 calories, eaten at one or two meals can result in new fat accumulation, the same 1500 calories spread out in six small meals, with two or three hour intervals, will not only fail to add weight, but may actually result in a weight loss!

4. Do not mix raw fruits and raw vegetables in the same meal.

Raw vegetables and raw fruits require a totally different

enzyme combination for their effective digestion. Combining them in the same meal will, therefore, only lead to poor digestion and gas. This applies also to mixing of fruit and vegetable juices.

It is best to make one main meal of the day, preferably breakfast, a fruit meal, another a grain (cereal) meal, and the third, a vegetable meal.

The exceptions to this rule are lemon, papaya, and avocado. They can be used with any foods, although avocado (botanically a fruit) is best eaten with a vegetable meal.

5. When protein-rich foods are eaten with other foods, eat protein-rich foods first.

Proteins require a generous amount of hydrochloric acid in your stomach in order to be properly digested. When you fill your stomach with carbohydrate-rich foods, such as salads, which do not require hydrochloric acid for digestion, your stomach will not have much hydrochloric acid because it is not secreted by the glands of the stomach when carbohydrate foods are eaten. Then, if you eat your steak, omelette, beans and tortillas, cheese soufflé, fish, or other protein-rich food, it will remain largely undigested because of an insufficient amount of hydrochloric acid in the stomach.

Therefore, it is best to eat protein foods first, *on an empty stomach,* when the hydrochloric acid secretion will be generous; then possibly continue with carbohydrate-rich foods. In practical terms, this would mean: steak first, then salad! Now, this is contrary to the traditional American way of serving salad first, before the entreé. (I say "American way" because this is not customary in other countries.) But the proof of the pudding is in the eating—it works! Try it and see for yourself how your digestion will improve. From a hypoglycemic point of view, abiding by this rule of eating will help to slow down the carbohydrate assimilation.

6. Practice systematic undereating.

Systematic undereating is the *Number One* health and longevity secret, just as systematic overeating is one of the main causes of disease and premature aging as well as one of the major contributing factors to the development of both hypoglycemia and diabetes.

My studies of centenarians around the world show that all of them have been moderate eaters throughout their lives. You never see an obese centenarian.

Food eaten in excess of actual body needs acts in the system as poison. It overloads the system with excessive sugar and contributes to disturbances in sugar metabolism. Overeating is particularly harmful for older people who are less active and have a slower metabolism. This is one of the main factors in geriatric diabetes, as well as in hypoglycemia, often both present in the same person.

The unbelievable truth is that *the less you eat, the less hungry you feel*, because the food is more effectively digested and better utilized.

WHAT ABOUT WATER

Before I complete this chapter on Optimum Nutrition for Hypoglycemia, I must cover the very important issue of your drinking needs. Water is very much a part of your nutrition. The minerals in natural waters have always played an important role in human nutrition. In fact, after millions of years of drinking naturally mineralized water from springs, rivers, lakes, and wells, our body has become dependent on mineral supplies from the water we drink.

Unfortunately, many have been confused on this issue by some misled or misinformed writers, who claim that the inorganic minerals in natural waters are harmful and cannot be utilized by our bodies. Because of such unsubstantiated notions, some people now drink nothing but distilled water, which is totally mineral-free.

Reliable world-wide research on water—and it is a massive research—shows that the above notion is completely false. The truth is that:

1. Minerals in natural waters are well digested and assimilated by the body. Although they are *inorganic* (as opposed to *organic* minerals that are in foods), they are chelated by the body in the intestinal tract and, thus, changed into organic form.

2. The statistics from United States and England, where extensive studies were made, show that wherever people drink naturally hard (heavy mineralized) water, they have less heart disease, less diabetes, less hardening of the arteries, less osteoporosis, and less tooth decay.

There is another good reason why hypoglycemics, especially, should make sure that they have the benefit of naturally mineralized water. Natural water is one of the few good natural sources of chromium, a trace mineral that is vitally involved in proper sugar metabolism. Chromium is a co-factor with insulin, and is essential not only for the effective utilization of sugar, but also for cholesterol metabolism and even the synthesis of protein.

Unfortunately, much of our tap water today is too polluted to be considered safe for drinking. Most stores are now selling pure or purified bottled water, or even spring water. I recommend this kind of water for drinking and cooking. If, for some reason, you are not able to get good, naturally-mineralized water and must rely on distilled water, you can improve its health-protective and nutritional quality by adding 2 tbsp. of plain sea water for each half gallon (or 1 tsp. of sea water concentrate). Bottled sea water is often sold in health food stores. There is also a concentrated mineral liquid supplement made in Utah from Salt Lake water; it is

sold in health food stores and can be added to distilled water.
Prolonged use of distilled water, unless it is re-mineralized
as suggested above, may result in severe mineral
deficiencies in the system since it tends to leach minerals out
of the body.

Suggested Menu
for the
Hypoglycemic

On the basis of the information presented in the previous Chapter, I will now outline a suggested menu for a daily diet. Please keep in mind the following:

1. The Menu consists of three main meals.

2. Between meals, throughout the day, the hypoglycemic should eat 3–4 snacks. Choose any one of the recommended snacks for *"Midmorning."*

3. For each main meal, I will list several *Choices.* "Choice 1" is the most ideal and the one I recommend. The following Choices are listed in order of preference—the higher on the list, the more desirable.

4. Since we are all different, with a different biochemical makeup and a different degree of sugar metabolism disorder, feel free to select the choices you desire most and those with which you feel best.

5. Breakfast and lunch are interchangeable; lunch and dinner are also interchangeable. If lunch suggestions are chosen for breakfast, then breakfast choices should be used for lunch—and vice versa. The same applies to lunch-dinner interchanges.

6. In most cases, I do not specify the quantity of food to be consumed. Generally speaking, you should eat enough to satisfy your hunger. However, if overweight is your prob-

lem, eat smaller portions. Regulate the quantity of food by the weight you wish to attain and/or maintain.

7. All vitamin and mineral supplements should be taken with the three main meals. See Chapter 9 for special supplements for hypoglycemia.

8. No liquids (water, juice, tea) should be consumed with meals, unless so specified.

UPON ARISING

Choice 1: Glass of pure spring water to which add freshly-squeezed juice of ½ lime, or ¼ lemon, or ½ grapefruit, or 1 orange.

Choice 2: Cup of freshly made herb tea (see Chapter 10 for suggested herbs for hypoglycemia). Tea can be sweetened with ½ tsp. natural, raw honey. Severe cases with extreme sensitivity to concentrated sweets should omit honey.

Choice 3: Glass of pure water with tsp. apple cider vinegar.

Choice 4: Glass of special drink. This choice is suggested for severe cases who feel weak and hungry in the morning and need an extra support.

Special Hypoglycemia Drink

1 cup raw, whole, unpasteurized milk
  or: 1 cup kefir, yogurt, or other soured milk
  or: ½ cup fresh fruit juice and ½ cup water
½ small banana or equivalent of other fresh fruit
  (omit if fruit juice is used)
1 tsp. dry skim milk powder
1 tsp. brewer's yeast powder
1 tsp. flax seeds, sesame seeds, or chia seeds.

Place all ingredients in a blender and run on high until seeds are liquified. Drink slowly or eat with a spoon.

MORNING WALK

If your work and life-style schedule permits, you should have a brisk one-half to one hour walk every morning after your morning drink. If you don't think you have the time, just go to bed an hour earlier, get up one hour earlier, and *make the time.* Get into the habit of walking every morning, it is absolutely imperative for your health. Remember, you cannot just eat your way to health (see Chapter 14 for the importance of exercise and fresh air).

Adjust the speed of your walk to your level of energy and physical condition. Slow walking is okay. Brisk walking is better. Intermittent walking and jogging is best. If you feel tired, stop and rest, then continue.

The longer you can spend for the morning walking routine, the better. You may take an apple with you and eat it while you rest or nibble on it as you walk. But, walk you must if you wish to restore buoyant health!

If you have the time, stop in the middle of the walk and do your favorite calisthenics: bending, stretching, rotating, hopping . . . whatever. Do some deep breathing exercises, too.

If possible, get out of the city and go to the countryside for your morning walk. Perhaps you can drive out to the beach or to the woods. But even around the block is better than nothing. Choose streets that are not heavily trafficked to avoid smog.

If you have a garden, one hour of hard gardening work in the morning will be a good substitute for walking.

Upon returning from your long walk or garden work, and after a shower to wash the perspiration away, you are now, *but not before,* ready for your breakfast!

BREAKFAST

Choice 1:   Fresh fruit *in season:* an apple; or an orange; or ½ banana; or ½ grapefruit; or slice of fresh pineapple; or 1 cup fresh cherries or strawberries—whatever is available. Fruit should be, preferably, organically grown (buy from your health food store, or from a grower you know, or grow your own). Remember: the sweeter the fruit, the less you eat. You may have more than one kind of fruit, but let your body decide on the quantity. The best apples for the hypoglycemic are: pippins, northern spy, granny's.

Cup of yogurt, kefir, or soured milk, preferably made from goat's milk (see Recipes, Chapter 13).

Handful of raw nuts, such as almonds, or a tablespoon of flaxseed, chia seed, sesame seed, or pumpkin seed. Nuts and seeds can be ground in a seed grinder and sprinkled over fresh salad or yogurt.

Instead of yogurt or other soured milk, ½ cup of homemade cottage cheese, *kvark,* can be substituted (see Chapter 13 for Recipe). Ricotta is also a possibility.

Choice 2:   Cup sprouted wheat or other sprouted seeds.

1 glass kefir, yogurt, or other soured milk.

Choice 3:   Cup cooked cereal: millet, buckwheat or oats (see Chapter 13 for Recipes and Instructions). Millet is the best cereal for hypoglycemics.

1 tsp. olive or sesame seed oil, poured over

cereal when served. *Or:* 1 pat of sweet butter.

1 glass fresh, raw, unpasteurized milk, preferably goat's milk (sold in some health food stores).

Homemade apple sauce can be used on cereal, if desired (see Chapter 13 on how to make apple sauce without a sweetener).

Choice 4:   2–3 buckwheat pancakes (see Chapter 13 for Recipe).

1 glass fresh raw milk.

1–2 tbsp. homemade applesauce.

Choice 5:   Cup of raw, uncooked, rolled oats.

1 glass raw unpasteurized milk.

2 tbsp. homemade applesauce.

Choice 6:   1 or 2 eggs, soft boiled. Another way (the best way) to prepare eggs: separate the egg yolk from the white; poach the white; then scramble eggs at the table by mixing raw egg yolks with cooked whites.

1 slice whole grain bread, made without sugar. Rye bread is preferred. (See Chapter 13 for Recipes.)

1 pat fresh butter.

1 glass fresh, raw milk, or 1 cup herb tea.

MID-MORNING SNACK

Choice 1:   1 tbsp. ground flax seed, sesame seed, chia seed, or pumpkin seed, mixed with ½ glass water, or herb tea, or kefir. Eat slowly with a spoon and chew well.

Choice 2: 5–10 raw almonds, or equivalent of other raw, unroasted nuts.

Choice 3: 1 piece fresh fruit. Best fruits: sour apples, pears, cherries, pineapple, papaya, melons.

Choice 4: 1 slice cheddar, Swiss, or other natural cheese. *Or:* ½ cup cottage cheese, or kvark cheese, or ricotta cheese.

A half apple or other fresh fruit may be eaten with cheese.

Choice 5: ½ large avocado or 1 small avocado.

Choice 6: Special Hypoglycemia Drink (see Choice 4 "UPON ARISING").

ONE HOUR BEFORE LUNCH

1 tbsp. brewer's yeast powder, fortified with B_{12}.

¼ tsp. bone meal powder (or 1 calcium lactate tablet).

½ glass freshly squeezed grapefruit juice or pineapple juice.

Mix well and eat with a spoon. If the mixture is too thick, dilute with water. Make sure the yeast you use is labeled "brewer's yeast"; health food stores sell it. If fresh grapefruit or pineapple juice is not available, kefir or canned grapefruit or pineapple juice can be substituted. Make sure it is a pure *juice*, without added sugar, not a *juice drink*, which is a synthetic imitation loaded with sugar and artificial flavoring and colorings—shun it as poison, which it, in truth, is.

LUNCH

Choice 1: Bowl of cooked whole-grain cereal. The choice of: millet, buckwheat, oats, 5-grain cereal. (See Chapter 13 for Recipes and instructions how to prepare cereals.) Millet and buckwheat cereals are best for the hypoglycemic.

1 glass fresh, raw, unpasteurized milk, preferably goat's milk.

1 tbsp. cold-pressed olive oil, or cold-pressed sesame seed oil. Oil can be substituted for by 1 or 2 pats of high quality butter. (Buy your oils and butter at health food stores.)

Choice 2: ½ large fresh avocado.

Small vegetable salad or ½ glass fresh vegetable juice can be eaten with avocado.

Choice 3: Any of the Breakfast Choices, if not eaten for breakfast.

Choice 4: Vegetable salad meal (see Dinner menu).

Choice 5: Bowl of freshly prepared vegetable, mushroom, pea or bean soup, or any other cooked or steamed vegetable dish, such as vegetable stew, zucchini, squash, green beans, corn, etc.

1 slice whole-grain bread.

1 slice natural cheese.

1 pat raw butter.

Choice 6: For Mexican food lovers: beans and corn tortillas with fresh tomato, onion, garlic, and chili salsa.

Choice 7: ½ cup drained, canned salmon, sardines, or tuna fish. Small vegetable salad.

MID-AFTERNOON SNACK

Two or two-and-one-half hours after lunch, repeat one of the Mid-morning Choices for a snack.

ONE HOUR BEFORE DINNER

Choice 1: ½ glass (2–3 oz.) freshly made vegetable juice, preferably Formula-H, Green Juice Cocktail (see Chapter 13 for Recipe and Instructions).

Choice 2: Same as "One Hour Before Lunch".

DINNER

Choice 1: Large bowl fresh green vegetable salad. Use any available vegetables, but especially avocados, cucumbers, tomatoes, mushrooms, onions, and garlic. Go easy on carrots. Greens of all kinds are best. Jerusalem artichokes, raw, are an excellent addition to salad.

Any available sprouts: mung beans, alfalfa, soybeans or wheat sprouts.

For salad dressing: fresh lime or lemon juice, or apple cider vinegar, mixed with olive or sesame seed oil, with natural herbs and spices, such as dill, cayenne, garlic powder, kelp, etc. Pinch of sea salt or herbal seasoning —sold at health food stores.

Choice of cooked, prepared vegetable dish: green beans, zucchini, squash, vegetable soup, vegetable stew, steamed vegetables, pea soup, beans or bean soup, mushrooms or mushroom soup, 1 baked or boiled potato, or yam.

1 slice whole-grain bread (see Chapter 13 for Recipe).

1-2 pats fresh raw butter.

1 slice cheddar or other natural cheese, or ½ cup kvark cheese (see Recipes).

1 glass kefir, yogurt, acidophilus milk, piimä, or any other soured milk.

Choice 2: Any of the Lunch Choices, if fresh vegetable salad is eaten at lunch.

EVENING SNACK

Choice 1: 1 cup yogurt or kefir with ½ tbsp. brewer's yeast.

Choice 2: 1 glass fresh, warmed milk with 1 plain whole-grain rye cracker.

Choice 3: 1 apple, eat slowly and chew well.

Choice 4: 1 cup warm herb tea with 2 tbsp. milk added.

1 rye cracker.

Vital points to remember

1. The above Menu is only a very general outline, a skeleton, around which you must build your own personalized diet, depending on the severity of your condition and your individual needs and lifestyle. I recommend following this Menu and dietary outline as closely as possible, but certain modifications and changes are allowed to make it adaptable to your specific requirements, food preferences, living conditions, ethnic background and customs, the climate where you live, the availability of foods recommended, etc.

2. The main feature of the Diet is that it provides 6–8 meals a day—a constant, uninterrupted supply of natural sources of sugar. As the condition improves and you can extend longer and longer the periods of time that you can function normally without food, you may skip some of the between-meal snacks.

3. In some extreme cases of hypoglycemia, the patient may be super-sensitive, even allergic, to practically all concentrated carbohydrates and sugars. If this applies to you, you must modify my diet to exclude, at least initially until your condition improves, all sweet fruits, honey, sweet juices, starchy vegetables, and even grains (except millet). See the Table of Food Composition at the end of the book and select vegetables and other foods that are low in starches. After following this diet for some time, the body will be more and more "de-sensitized" and more able to tolerate natural carbohydrate foods. When the hypoglycemic is actually allergic to carbohydrates, carbohydrate tolerance must be built up gradually. The emphasis at such a stage must be on natural protein-rich foods, such as almonds, millet, buckwheat, pumpkin seeds, sesame seed, milk, natural cheese, cottage cheese or kvark, yogurt or kefir, and possibly eggs or fish, if desired. But remember, even the most severe hypoglycemic needs some carbohydrate in the diet. This fact has now been recognized even by the hard-core high-protein advocates.[7,49] Carbohydrates are actually needed both for proper metabolism of proteins and for the synthesis of proteins in the liver. Carbohydrates are also needed to prevent or decrease the destruction of body protein and prevent acidosis.[50]

4. When hypoglycemics travel and must eat at restaurants, following a strict diet presents a problem. Actually, it is not as difficult a problem as you may think. Most roadside coffee-houses still serve old-fashioned oatmeal cereal for breakfast. With a glass of milk and a couple of pats of butter,

oatmeal can make an excellent breakfast. Eggs in shell is the other natural food that is available at most restaurants at any time of the day. Two eggs, soft boiled, with a slice of rye bread, can be used for lunch or dinner. Of course hypoglycemics should have a supply of raw nuts (almonds) when they travel.

5. Once the condition is corrected and the function of the adrenal system and pancreas is normalized, I suggest that you continue with the Optimum Diet, as outlined in this book, to prevent relapse. This diet will not only prevent or correct hypoglycemia, but it will build a higher level of general health, helping you to avoid most of our degenerative diseases as well. It would certainly be unwise, after health has been improved and hypoglycemia corrected, to go back to the old ways of eating and living—the ways that were largely responsible for the development of disease in the first place.

Special Supplements for Hypoglycemia

The hypoglycemia diet should be supplemented with the following adult daily doses of vitamins, minerals, and other supplements. These supplements have been found in research and clinical experience to have a favorable supportive and therapeutic effect in the management of hypoglycemia.

Taking into consideration the biochemical individuality of each patient, the dosage needed or tolerated by different individuals may vary considerably. This will depend on the severity of the condition, the patient's nutritional status, age, medical history, his ability to digest and utilize foods, his level of physical and mental stress, his environmental situation, etc. Therefore, it must be understood that the suggested dosage is only given as a general guidance. Only you and your doctor can know what will be the most suitable dosage *for you.*

VITAMINS AND SUPPLEMENTS (daily)

Vitamin C—2,000 mg. to 3,000 mg.

Vitamin C increases the body's tolerance to sugars and carbohydrates and helps to normalize sugar metabolism. It is also a potent detoxifier and improves the adrenal hormonal output. The best form of supplementary vitamin C is natural vitamin C-complex with bioflavonoids.[7,9,56]

B-complex, 100% natural, from yeast concentrate—4 to 6 tablets

Vitamins from B-complex are known to be anti-stress vitamins. They are also involved in sugar metabolism, normalizing sugar levels. B-vitamin deficiencies can disturb the carbohydrate metabolism by disrupting normal liver functions. Make sure that the brand you buy is 100% natural, since most B-complex formulations, even those sold in health food stores, are synthetic. The high potency isolated B vitamins, which are also recommended for hypoglycemics, will have to be synthetic, but the B-complex supplement must be all natural.[9]

Vitamin B6—50 mg. to 100 mg.

Vitamin B_6 regulates the balance between the minerals sodium and potassium in the body, which is of tremendous importance to all body functions, including sugar metabolism. Vitamin B_6 also helps in building up adrenals which are often exhausted in hypoglycemics. This vitamin is involved in energy production and can help prevent obesity in those who are predisposed to it, as are many hypoglycemics. The deficiency of B_6 can cause damage to the pancreas.[9,50]

Pantothenic acid—100 mg. to 200 mg.

Pantothenic acid is primarily an anti-stress factor. It stimulates the adrenal glands and increases production of adrenal hormones. Severe deficiency of this vitamin may cause low blood sugar as well as low blood pressure. The deficiency of pantothenic acid is specifically associated with a rapid drop in sugar level.[9,50]

Vitamin E, natural, mixed tocopherols—600 I.U. to 1,200 I.U. (specified in terms of d-alpha tocopherol potency)

Vitamin E improves the oxygenation of cells. It is of specific importance at times when sugar levels are low. The deficiency of vitamin E may contribute to the degeneration of the adrenal cortex.[50] Vitamin E protects the pituitary and the adrenal hormones from destruction by oxygen.[57] The dosage of vitamin E must be determined individually, since some hypoglycemics feel overstimulated by large dosages. Start with 100 I.U. a day and increase gradually.

Vitamin B12—25 mcg. to 50 mcg.

Vitamin B_{12} is helpful in regeneration of the liver which is often toxic or overstressed in the hypoglycemic.[50] Brewer's yeast, fortified with B_{12}, is the best food source.

Magnesium-calcium supplement—2 to 3 tablets (dolomite or other magnesium-calcium supplements can be used)

Magnesium and calcium are needed to balance the excess of phosphorus in brewer's yeast, which is one of the most important supplementary foods for hypoglycemics. Magnesium is involved in sugar metabolism and energy production. Calcium is vital to all body functions, but especially in the proper utilization of other minerals as well as of vitamins D, A, and C.

Bone-meal—3 tablets or ½ tsp. powder

Bone-meal is a good natural source of organic minerals and trace elements. The best kind of bone meal supplement is raw, unheated, and preferably imported from South America (less contaminated).

Potassium citrate—300 mg. to 500 mg. (or potassium chloride up to 200 mg.)

Potassium is important for proper sugar metabolism. Low levels of blood potassium may cause a drop in blood sugar. All stress contributes to potassium loss, which results in dangerously excessive levels of sodium in the tissues, with accompanying edema.

Vitamin A & D supplement—1 or 2 capsules (10,000 units of A and 400 units of D per capsule)

Both vitamins are vital in virtually all body functions, but specifically in effective mineral assimilation and synergistic action of other vitamins.

Multiple mineral and trace element formula—1 to 2 tablets

This must be a comprehensive mineral and trace element formula, which includes, but is not limited to, the following trace elements which are specifically involved in healthy sugar metabolism: iron, zinc, copper, chromium, selenium, manganese, and molybdenum. Health food stores carry several brands. The broad spectre, low-potency formula, possibly in a chelated form, would be the best.

Brewer's yeast—3 to 4 tbsp. of powder or an equivalent in tablets

The detailed description of the reasons for taking yeast by hypoglycemics can be found in Chapter 7.

Lecithin—2 tsp. of granules

Lecithin is important for proper fat metabolism and for

the healthy function of the brain, nervous system, and sex glands.

Kelp—2 tablets or ½ tsp. of granules

Kelp is a good natural source of iodine and other trace elements.

Sea water—1 to 2 tbsp. a day or ½ tsp. of concentrate

Sea water is a good natural source of trace elements. It can be used to re-mineralize distilled water.

Special notes on taking vitamins and supplements

1. The above dosages are calculated for *adults.* Children, age 10 to 15, should take ¼ of the adult dose; age 15 to 18—½ dose. Children, age 15 to 18, should take no more than 200 I.U. of vitamin E; if they are under the age of 15, none.

2. Take all vitamins and supplements for two to three months. After an interval of 6 to 8 weeks, the supplementary program can be repeated.

3. The supplements should be divided equally and taken with the three main meals.

4. An exception to the previous note: If the trace element formula contains *iron,* it should not be taken at the time when vitamin E is taken. In such a case, it will be best to take all vitamin E in the morning, and the iron-containing formula in the evening. Vitamin E and the *supplementary* iron are antagonistic to each other (*natural* iron in food does not interfere with vitamin E.).

5. All the suggested vitamins, minerals, and other supplements are available from health food stores, where you can also get advice on the most suitable brands.

6. If at all possible, use only 100 percent natural brands.

7. If your condition is serious and taking vitamins on your own doesn't seem to help, it would be wise to consult an experienced physician or nutritionist who can tailor the supplementary program to fit your specific personal needs and requirements. For the way to find a nutritionally-oriented doctor, see Chapter 1.

8. Hypoglycemic patients with an overweight problem should double the dosage of B6, kelp, and lecithin, and should also take apple cider vinegar with meals. Obviously, they should also eat smaller portions and do more exercise.

9. If you suffer from digestive disorders, gas, and assimilation problems (especially if you are over fifty) you should take, in addition to the above supplements, 1 or 2 tablets of multiple digestive enzyme formula after each main meal. Try to get one comprehensive digestive formula which contains hydrochloric acid, pancreatic enzymes, pepsin, papaine, ox bile, lipase, bromelain, etc.

10. Some doctors use injections of complete adrenocortical extract (ACE) intramuscularly (in oil), or intravenously (aquaeous ACE), in addition to a nutritional program and the usual supplements. Dr. Alan Nittler, one of the leading experts on the treatment of hypoglycemia, uses the following formula:[51]

Aquaeous adrenocortical extract:	1,000 mcgm.
Vitamin B_{12} (cyanocobalamine):	1,000 mcgm.
Vitamin C (ascorbic acid):	250 mg.
Vitamin B_6 (pyridoxine):	100 mg.
Calcium glycerophosphate: (Calphosan®)	2 cc.
Dilute hydrochloric acid (1:1,000):	10 cc.

Your doctor can advise you on the need and suitability of this formula for you.

11. Some doctors, in addition to my diet and the usual supplements, use protomorphogens (see report from Dr. Gabriel K. Cousens, M.D. in Chapter 12). Protomorphogens are natural animal raw gland tissues. They come in tablet form and are best taken orally by dissolving the tablets in the mouth, whereby the active factors may be absorbed by special pathways through the membranes of the mouth. This prevents the destruction of the active factors in protomorphogens by the digestive juices in the stomach. Again, your doctor will be the one to advise you if you should use protomorphogens.

Special Herbs
for Hypoglycemia

Herbs have been used as healing agents since the beginning of time by every race upon the earth. Traditionally, people in every corner of this planet possessed remarkable knowledge of the medicinal value of certain roots, barks, seeds, and plants that grew in their environment. This knowledge was handed down from one generation to the next.

Later, when primitive medicine was replaced by modern pharmaceuticals, much of the medical pharmocopoeia that doctors used was made up of botanical medicines: herbs, roots, etc.

In studying herbal manuals from many countries during the last forty years, I have found herbal medicines listed for every conceivable ailment or health disorder, except one: hypoglycemia! This is because hypoglycemia is a relatively new disease, recognized as such only in the last couple of decades—and most herbal manuals were written before this time. Even one of the currently most popular books on herbal therapy, BACK TO EDEN, does not list hypoglycemia or low blood sugar.

Consequently, discouraged, but not willing to give up, convinced that there must be effective herbs even for hypoglycemia as there is for every other ailment, I was forced to do my own research and investigation of the subject. My intimate knowledge of Mexican herbology was of special help. In Mexico, botanical medicine is highly advanced and has survived until present times in spite of the availability of chemical drugs. The knowledge of herbal medicine and its traditional uses is carefully preserved by skilled herbalists; and botanical medicine is even taught in some Mexican universities.

On the basis of my research, I have found the following several herbs to be beneficial in hypoglycemia.

- **Juniper cedar berries** (Juniperus Sabina Pinaceae), have a nourishing, regulating, and stimulating effect on the pancreas and are useful in the treatment of both diabetes and hypoglycemia.[9]

- **Capalchi, or Copalquin** (Croton Niveus), also known as **Quina Blanca** in Mexico. It grows in Mexico, Central and South America, and the West Indies. It has a stabilizing effect on blood sugar levels and is therapeutically effective for both hypoglycemia and diabetes.[52]

- **Licorice root** (Glycyrrhiza Glabra) is a powerful builder of adrenals and one of the most important herbs for the hypoglycemic.[9,53]

- **Mexican wild yam** (Dioscorea Villosa) has a beneficial regulating effect on endocrine hormonal imbalances, especially on the function of the adrenals. It also aids in the synthesis of sex hormones.[53]

- **Golden seal** (Hydrastis) is another outstanding herb that can help not only in normalizing blood sugar levels, but also is one of the most versatile herbal remedies for a variety of disorders, specifically nervous problems, female disorders, prostate problems, lymphatic disorders, and digestive problems.[54] Golden seal must be used in very small quantities.

- **Lobelia** (Lobelia Inflata) is also helpful in supporting the adrenal and liver functions.[52]

- **Other beneficial herbs,** which are of more general value, but are also useful for hypoglycemia, are: dandelion, garlic, horsetail, American helebore, chicory, wahoo, and cornsilk. They stimulate and improve the function of the entire digestive and metabolic systems, which include liver, pancreas, stomach, and gall bladder.[54] Dandelion (root and leaves) is a powerful detoxifier of the liver and can help to normalize liver function.[9] Garlic is also an excellent detoxifier; it improves the general metabolism and has a stimulating effect on the liver, the circulation, and the nervous system. It also strengthens the body's defenses against allergens—hypoglycemics often suffer from allergy. Those who cannot eat fresh garlic for social reasons (odor), can use an excellent new *odorless* garlic product, *Kyolic*, developed in Japan. It is sold in most health food stores. If unavailable, write to the company: Wakunaga of America Co., P.O. Box 22280, Honolulu, Hawaii 96822.

Where to get these herbs

Most of the above mentioned herbs are sold in health food stores, either packaged in dry form, capsulated, or sometimes tableted. If your store doesn't carry them, try herb houses—see your telephone directory for addresses or check the advertisers in such publications as *Let's Live* Magazine or *Prevention* (both also sold at health food stores).

A few of the mentioned herbs are rare and difficult to get. Juniper cedar berries and Copalquin are often hard to locate. Try several herb companies.

How to use herbs

The most common way to use herbs is in the form of herb teas, or what is professionally known as *infusions.*

Here is how you make herb teas:

Take one to two tsp. of dried herbs (or the powder of 2–3 capsules) to a cup of water; or, take 1 oz. of the dried herb to 1 pint of water, if a larger quantity is desired. Boil the water. Place the herbs in a cup or other container and pour the boiling water over the herbs. Cover and let steep for 15 minutes. Stir, let settle, strain, and let cool down to a drinkable temperature—never drink the tea boiling hot! There is no wisdom in curing hypoglycemia and dying of stomach cancer, which excessive drinking of scalding hot liquids surely can cause. Note: never boil herb teas or even simmer them, just pour hot water over the herbs and let steep.

If you use capsulated or tableted herbs, crush the tablets or open the capsules, discarding the gelatin capsules, and pour boiling water over them. Let steep 5 to 10 minutes. Stir and drink; no need for straining.

The best time to drink herb teas is the first thing in the morning, two hours before or after a meal, and before going to bed.

It is always best to prepare fresh tea every time. At any rate, do not make more tea than can be used in one day.

The best utensils to make herb teas are glass, pyrex, stoneware, or stainless steel. Do not use aluminum.

11

Doctors' Report

At the time this is written, the new diet for hypoglycemia as presented in this book is being used by many physicians. I have asked four doctors, who have used my diet extensively, to share their experiences with the readers of this book. The communications received from the doctors are reprinted below in their entirety.

1. A Letter from Bill Gray, M.D.

Dr. Gray is a member of the International Academy of Biological Medicine, and practices in Mill Valley, California. He specializes in biological medicine, nutrition, and homeopathy.

Dear Dr. Airola:

I will be happy to share my experiences in the treatment of hypoglycemia with the readers of your new book.

Your approach to nutrition has almost infallibly cured hypoglycemia in my experience. For the first two years of practice, I treated hypoglycemia patients with the high-protein diet. I found their hypoglycemic symptoms moderately well controlled, but the patients felt much worse. They developed low energy levels, headaches, skin problems, arthritis, and various digestive disturbances. An interesting observation that I have not yet been able to explain: People on high-protein diets have their hypoglycemic symptoms controlled, but they have worse reactions to smaller amounts of sugar. Whereas they would have a full-blown reaction to a chocolate cake in the past, they would react just as fully to the sugar coating on a vitamin pill while on the high-protein diet.

After learning your common-sense approach to diet, the entire issue of hypoglycemia became clear to me. After all, the human race has evolved on a basic, natural-carbohydrate oriented diet since the advent of agriculture about 12,000 years ago. Our metabolisms, therefore, are best adjusted to a low-protein, high-natural-carbohydrate diet: grains, seeds, nuts, vegetables, fruits, and some dairy products. In the past few hundred years, the advent of wealthy industrialized society has taken foods customarily accessory to the diet, and made them central to the diet, i.e., sugar, refined flour, meat, fish, and fowl. This is how foods designed to be accessory to our metabolism have overloaded our metabolisms, and thus produced symptoms of sugar metabolism disorder.

In my opinion, hypoglycemia is *not a disease.* It is merely a set of symptoms caused by substances not fitted to the metabolism. If the human race had introduced arsenic into the diet, the symptoms coming from the poisoning would not be a disease. The solution would not be to introduce another abnormal substance into the diet to control the symptoms; it would be to simply return to the natural diet, free from any abnormal substances.

Hypoglycemia is the result of ingesting small-molecule carbohydrates, causing a sudden flood of glucose into the bloodstream. This occurs because such molecules are absorbed nearly instantaneously across the membranes of the mouth and stomach. Normally, carbohydrate molecules, from natural carbohydrate-rich foods, are slowly broken down from their long chains into small molecules and ultimately absorbed slowly in the small intestine. The process of refining carbohydrates breaks them into small molecules; the subsequent flood of glucose into the bloodstream causes a tremendous reaction of the pancreas, adrenals, liver, and possibly of other organs, to restore the blood sugar to normal. After continued exposure, this reaction itself becomes abnormal, resulting in the symptoms of hypoglycemia.

The standard approach is to use a high-protein diet. Protein molecules are long-chain molecules which are slowly broken down and slowly absorbed. Each unit of the protein can be converted to glucose, and because this is a gradual process, the blood sugar is stabilized without sudden swings. Unfortunately, each unit of the protein molecule also contains a nitrogen unit which must be separated from the carbohydrate portion and then excreted via the liver and kidney. Since the body's metabolism has evolved to handle only 20–25 grams of protein a day, a diet containing 60, 80, even 120 grams of protein puts a great stress on the system. It requires great energy to excrete the nitrogen toxins. The result is fatigue, and the toxins that are not excreted cause a wide variety of symptoms themselves harmful to the health.

A classic case example: A man of 30 complained of hypoglycemia for over five years. The diagnosis was confirmed by two 5-hour glucose tolerance tests spaced years apart. Finally, he saw a physician (a friend of mine) who prescribed a high-protein meal every two hours. The patient followed it strictly. His hypoglycemia symptoms cleared up, but he became so fatigued and plagued with headaches that he could make it to his job as a truck driver only half the time. After eating, he felt so poorly, that it became clear to him that that was doing him harm. He reduced the number of meals, but stuck to high protein foods; he felt a little better, but was still largely crippled. Finally, after trying the diet for eight months, he came down with the flu. Despite good care, he had not recovered from the flu after three months. I concluded that his problem stemmed more from protein toxicity than from hypoglycemia. I put him on a 10-day fast, then on your high-natural-carbohydrate diet with only three meals a day. He felt absolutely well after a few days on the fast, and he continued to feel well thereafter. As a matter of fact, from the time of the fast on, he was able to work full time, run 5–6 miles daily, and take karate lessons three times weekly. His energy was good, he had no headaches or "flu" symptoms, and no return of his hypoglycemia symptoms.

I hope these comments will be useful to you and your readers. Good luck on your much needed book.

2. A Letter From Gabriel K. Cousens, M.D.

Dr. Cousens is on the Medical Advisory Board of the International Academy of Biological Medicine, and has a private practice in Elk, California. He specializes in biological medicine, nutrition, herbology, and the total life-styling.

Dear Dr. Airola:

I have followed twenty-five patients with hypoglycemia, using a low-protein, high-natural-carbohydrate diet, from six to thirteen months. I have attained good results with your diet plus protomorphogens. I found the results supportive to the conclusions that your diet is a key to healing in hypoglycemia and health in general.

Enclosed are a Basic Data Sheet for twenty-five patients, a Summary, a Discussion, and five detailed case histories. I hope they are useful to you in your book.

BASIC DATA SHEET
(see the next two pages)

(A Study of 25 cases of hypoglycemia treated by Gabriel K. Cousens, M.D.).

ABBREVIATIONS:

"D" or "Diet" = Airola Diet

"P" or "Proto" = Protomorphogens

"Months" = Time it took to reach a certain level of healing.

Patient No.	No Change	0–19% Improvement	20–49% Improvement	50–79% Improvement	80–94% Improvement (without symptoms on diet, but symptoms return in hours to 3 days when off diets)	95–99% Improvement (almost totally healed)	Completely Healed
1					4 months D+P	8 months D+P	
2						5 months D+P	
3						12 months D	12 months D +3 months D+P +5 months maintenance D.
4				6 months D (then got pregnant)			
5						10 months D	
6					3 months D+P	7 months D+P	
7				6 months D	6 months D +2 months D+P		
8					4 months D+P		8 months D+P plus 5 months without relapse on D.
9					6 months D+P	13 months D+P	
10		5 months 20% D				9 months D	
11					3 months D 5 months P	10 months D	
12		4 months D+P		7 months D+P	3 months D 5 months P		
13						11 months D 2 months D+P	

Patient No.	No Change	0-19% Improvement	20-49% Improvement	50-79% Improvement	80-94% Improvement (without symptoms on diet, but symptoms return in hours to 3 days when off diets)	95-99% Improvement (almost totally healed)	Completely Healed
14						13 months D	
15			7 months D (then off Diet)	2 months D			
16				4 months D			4 months D +7 months D+P (Total 11 months)
17				2 months D+P			7 months D+P
18				8 months D			8 months D +3 months D+P (Total 11 months)
19	(Suffering from subacute infective hepatitis)		2 months D+P	9 months D+P			
20						9 months D / 13 months D	
21						3 months D / 8 months D	
22		(patient suffers from mercury poisoning)			3 months D+P		
23	8 months D						
24					3 months D+P	4 months D+P	
25						5 months D+P .	

SUMMARY

25 subjects were followed for 6 months to 1 year or more on Airola Diet plus indicated supplementary minerals, vitamins, herbs, and protomorphogens. Of these:

12 on diet alone, plus supplementary vitamins and minerals, and

13 on diet plus protomorphogens (prescribed for either pancreas, adrenal regeneration, or both). In the second category, the subjects were often put on protomorphogens after reaching a stable diet. Previous clinical experience suggested that the protomorphogens without a proper diet did not seem effective.

On diet alone, 8.3% had 100% healings; 58% had 95%–99%, or almost healed; 8.3% had 80%–99% symptom removal and basic relief and stabilization; 16.6% had 50%–79% symptom relief; 8.3% had no change in symptoms. On diet plus protomorphogens, 38% had complete healing; 46% had 95%–99% healing; 15% had 50%–79% healing.

DISCUSSIONS

The categories used above have their own particular definitions:

100% healed means not only no symptoms whatsoever, but also sustained resiliency of a person's system when he goes off the diet for a period of time. It is usually marked by a clear improvement in life situation and confidence in body-endocrine integrity. These people could fast without any difficulty.

95%–99% healed means all or almost all the symptoms are gone, but that if the person went off the diet for four days to several weeks, symptoms would recur. These people still had difficulty fasting, but some could.

80%–94% healed means that most of the symptoms are relieved, the person's life is stabilized, but if he goes off the diet for more than a few days, symptoms recur.

50%–80% healing means that the person's life isn't entirely stabilized, and that only 50%–80% of the symptoms are relieved, or these symptoms are decreased in severity. If he goes off the diet, he has immediate difficulty.

20%–49% healing means some of the symptoms are lessened by that percentage.

"No improvement" speaks for itself. In this case, the person with no improvement also was being treated for mercury poisoning, with some overlapping symptoms.

My feeling for the overall picture is that the Airola Diet is very effective in healing hypoglycemia and that it is a very healthy diet in general, which people can maintain for the rest of their lives. On diet alone, approximately ¾ of the people had at least symptom removal to the point that hypoglycemia was no longer a significant, or even a minor factor affecting their lives. Only one person in all 25 cases did not improve. With diet alone, or with diet plus protomorphogens, ⁴/₅ of the people reached the point of being free from hypoglycemic symptoms.

A significant trend was that a good percentage of those who eventually obtained complete healing, went with diet alone only to category 95%–99%, and needed protomorphogens to obtain a complete recovery within a year's time. It isn't clear that if they had stayed on the diet alone for longer than 1⅓ years they could have reached the stage of complete recovery.

Most of the patients received a 5-hour glucose tolerance test, hair analysis, detailed clinical survey and history, and Ridler's test. Before the diagnosis was made, I observed a 100% correlation of positive glucose tolerance test with a positive hair analysis pattern, history, and Ridler's test.

Part way in the study, patients were given an option of taking or not taking a GTT. I made the ethical decision not to traumatize their nervous and endocrine systems with a GTT to determine if the person was healed. Instead, a subjective symptom rating form was given to each to be filled out during each follow-up visit, at which time they were interviewed about their hypoglycemia symptoms.

FIVE CASE HISTORIES
from Dr. Gabriel K. Cousens' Files

1. J. A., 36-year-old, white male

Without previous history of any major sickness, he developed a sudden onset of hypoglycemic symptoms one year after starting a high-vitamin, high-protein diet. It started at age 31, with feelings of panic, anxiety attacks, fear of dying. These attacks increased from one every 6 months to eventually 2 times per week. By this time, he had dizziness, fatigue, excessive anxiety, concentration fade-outs, low energy, craving for alcohol, fears, phobias, insomnia, and blurred vision.

In 1972, hypoglycemia was diagnosed by a glucose tolerance test. Blood glucose lows were down to 9 mg./100 ml. By this time, he had lost his job, and was suicidal. He tried a high-protein, multiple-meal diet. His weight dropped from 165 to 125 pounds, and he began to feel worse.

In 1974, he began seeing a psychoanalyst for his depression. He was also put on 7½ to 15 mg. valium for anxiety.

He came to me in May of 1975. He was put on the Airola Diet plus potassium, chromium, and manganese for these specific mineral deficiencies. Two months later, he began to experience more energy, absence of shaking spells, and some moderate relief of his extreme anxiety. He was only partially on the diet at this time. In four months, his anxiety decreased; he no longer was frightened by physical pain. Anxiety attacks, which had been 4–5 times per day were reduced to very mild states; panic attacks, or severe anxiety attacks, which occured twice a week, were down to once a month. At this point, diet was stable enough to begin the use of protomorphogens.

He was improving continuously during the next seven months, needing valium only occasionally. He began to talk more often about feeling good and enjoying life. The case is still in progress.

2. 52-year-old female, school teacher

Since childhood, she had symptoms of unexplained mood changes, irritability, anxiety, depression, concentration fadeouts, low energy, shakiness, trembling, sweats, craving for sweets. She had a positive glucose tolerance test. The blood tests also revealed hypokalemia (low potassium levels). After 3–4 months on the Airola diet, all symptoms disappeared except the weakness and tiredness, which disappeared also after increasing the potassium supplementation. Examinations 7 months and again 1 year later showed that she was completely healed. "I feel like a person reborn. I didn't realize how feeling 'well' really felt. I feel balanced, deeply serene, and happy," were her comments.

3. 24-year-old female

Previously in good health, she had a sudden attack of severe hypoglycemia, highlighted by two emergency room visits where blood sugar tests revealed hypoglycemia. On physical examination, tenderness over the pancreas was felt. In addition to shock syndrome, she experienced constant tiredness, unexplained mood changes, anxiety, cravings for sweets, lack of concentration, panicky feelings, and unwanted psychic experiences. She was unable to work, and her life was out of control. Her HOD test was 54 when we started her on the Airola Diet plus iron and potassium supplements. After two weeks, the HOD dropped to 7. Two months later, her symptoms began to fade to the point where she was stabilized. Protomorphogens were added after 2½ months, and she was 80%–94% healed by 5 months. After 7 months of treatment, she was 95%–99% healed, had a job, and was feeling well. Eleven months after treatment began, she seemed completely healed and very much in control of her life.

4. 25-year-old white female

She suffered from moderate symptoms of hypoglycemia, including generally decreased functioning, craving for sweets, unexplained anxiety, depression, mood changes, lack of concentration, drowsiness, periods of confusion, craving for alcohol. She was put on the Airola Diet. After 1 year, she became almost symptom-free and maintained it for another year of follow up.

5. 33-year-old white female

She had a 13-year history of symptoms of weakness on awakening, fatigue in the late morning and afternoons, and unexplained mood changes, anxiety, depression, lack of concentration, feelings of hunger, low energy, craving for alcohol, and difficulty working. Diagnosis of hypoglycemia was confirmed by glucose tolerance test. She was started on the Airola Diet, plus adrenal and pancreatic protomorphogens, as well as electrolyte supplements for a general metabolic imbalance, as suggested by hair analysis. A two-week rest from work was also prescribed so she could have a better opportunity to adhere to her new diet. She did well during the two weeks, but had symptom recurrance when she went back to work. But she progressivly improved, and seven months later she was completely symptom-free and her health was 100% restored.

3. A Letter from Michael B. Schachter, M.D., and David Sheinkin, M.D.

> Drs. Schachter and Sheinkin are members of the International Academy of Biological Medicine, and practice in Nyack, New York. They specialize in psychiatry, and nutritional counseling. Here is their report on the use of the Airola Diet in the treatment of hypoglycemia.

Dear Dr. Airola:

Since our medical education was carried out at top-notch U.S. medical schools, we were taught little about nutrition and did not know much about hypoglycemia. It was not until we had been in practice for 8–9 years that through a series of coincidences we became interested in nutrition and its application to health and prevention of illness. This resulted, among other things, in our becoming aware of the almost epidemic proportions of hypoglycemia and of the many-faceted symptoms it could present.

Our general treatment approach to hypoglycemia (keeping in mind that whatever treatment we use is always individualized and considered in context of the whole person) stresses (a) an appropriate diet, (b) nutritional supplementation, (c) an "avoid" list similar to the Airola "avoid" list published in *How To Get Well,* (d) avoidance of foods (otherwise healthful) to which the patient has a specific brain sensitivity, (e) consideration of A.C.E., (f) consideration of short wave therapy.

Initially, the diet we recommended was the traditionally accepted high-protein, low-carbohydrate diet. As we became increasingly aware, through the writings of Airola and others, of the disadvantages and dangers inherent in the long-term use of high-protein diets, we began recommending the Airola Diet. We have been doing so regularly for the past 2½–3 years.

We have found that for most patients, either diet (and indeed other specific diets such as the low-fat diet described by Pritiken) will help to control the low blood sugar condition equally well. There is a small group of patients who will do much better on one of these diets than they will on the other (of these, the majority will fare better on the Airola diet). We would estimate that in the past 3 years, we have treated 300 patients with hypoglycemia, utilizing the Airola Diet. Their success rate is about 75%. Most failures on this diet can be attributed to specific sensitivities the individual has to certain foods included in the diet. When these foods are eliminated, or the diet rotated, these individuals also do well on the Airola Diet.

If our only concern was controlling the hypoglycemia, then, for most patients, it would make little difference which diet was used. However, as our concern is with the *overall health* of the individual, and the long term maintenance of health, we definitely favor the Airola Diet. We believe the Airola Diet to be more of a natural diet (more in tune with man's natural way of eating) and one which can help to avoid many of the chronic and degenerative diseases which are more and more becoming associated with prolonged high-protein intake.

Michael B. Schachter, M.D.
David Sheinkin, M.D.

Hypoglycemics Speak...

I receive hundreds of unsolicited letters from hypo-glycemics who have tried my diet and then have felt moved to tell me of their experiences. Here are just a few of them. I am including them in the book hoping that they will be not only an inspiration, but a help to the reader in solving his own health problems.

The case of Ms. L. G., Maryland

Dear Dr. Airola:

I am a 32-year-old woman with hypoglycemia. For six-teen months I was on a basic high-protein, low carbohydrate diet. For the first six months I felt better, especially during the first few weeks, but then I started getting sicker and sicker, constantly eating for temporary relief. After four months of the high protein diet, I had gained 30 pounds and have never been able to lose it. At that time the doctor found that I had low, but not abnormally low, thyroid, and he put me on thyroid pills, one grain per day. The pills seemed to give me a little more energy, but I still was very fatigued and unable to work. At that time, my blood test for thyroid and adrenal glands was low, but within the normal range.

After sixteen months on the high protein diet, and after getting progressively worse, new blood tests showed that my adrenals, in the doctor's words, "had shrunk beyond help."

He said there was nothing he could do.

Then I started going to a chiropractor. He put me on Drenatrophin (an extract from beef adrenal tissue), 6 per day. They seemed to help a little, but I still had symptoms every day: tension in the forehead, fatigue, headaches, stomach pain, and extreme nervousness most of the time. He was also doing some spinal adjustments.

Five weeks ago I went on your diet, after reading about it in *Let's Live* Magazine. I noticed an immediate difference. No more stomach pains, which were more or less constant before. I took some digestive tablets, 5-grain diluted hydrochloric acid and 1-grain pepsin. This seemed to help alleviate the other symptoms, although they sometimes gave me diarrhea. But I am steadily progressing and feeling much better and am much less tired now that I have stopped eating all those proteins. For the first time I have hopes that with the help of your diet I will be able to lick the problem.

The case of Miss H., Florida

Dear Dr. Airola:

My daughter was recently diagnosed as having hypoglycemia. Her doctor told her only to eliminate sugar and eat cheese. After reading the section on hypoglycemia in your new book, HOW TO GET WELL, my daughter has begun your suggested diet and special supplements, and now—only two weeks later—she is a new person!

The case of Mrs. M. G., New York

Dear Dr. Airola:

I have been suffering from low blood sugar for as long as I remember, but I was diagnosed only 3 years ago. I have been to three doctors since, but they have not been able to help me. They all suggested a high-protein, low- (natural or otherwise) carbohydrate diet. I am also overweight, so I found it very difficult to try to relieve my symptoms and lose weight at the same time. And considering all the symptoms I had, I believe my case was severe.

After reading your articles on hypoglycemia, I started on your diet. I felt so much better right away. After about three months, most of the symptoms disappeared and I was even able to lose 12 pounds. I love eating the cereals you recommend and now eat meat only once a week. I carry nuts in my purse and nibble on them when I feel like it. I make my own kefir and love it. I also take all the vitamins you recommend. I haven't felt so strong and energetic since my teenage years.

The case of Mr. D. H., California

Dear Dr. Airola:

I started your hypoglycemia diet a year ago and, right away, I felt that it would be most helpful to me. For several years after first being exposed to "health foods", I was very confused. First, I went on an extremely high protein diet with lots of "fortified" milk and hardly any fruits or vegetables. I felt great for a year or so, but eventually got completely clogged up and full of mucus. My kidneys were sore, apparently from too much meat and raw eggs. Then, I switched to a totally opposite direction. I went on a mostly raw fruits diet to cleanse myself. I felt so rejuvenated, I couldn't believe it. But I kept wasting away and soon developed a taste for the junk foods that I used to like as a child.

When I tried your diet, however, it seemed to satisfy me completely and I have no more desire for sweets. Although I have been on it only a year, I can truthfully say that my low blood sugar is now, for the first time, completely under control. I feel stronger than I did on the fruitarian diet, and less toxic and filled with mucus than I did on the high-protein diet. I still have to eat every two hours or so, but eventually I hope to get along on a lesser number of meals. I am not taking any of the vitamins you recommend, being of the opinion that we should get vitamins and minerals from natural foods. Perhaps, with the supplements and vitamins, I would feel even better.

The case of Dr. T., California

Dear Dr. Airola:

After fifteen years of suffering with a series of harsh, but apparently unrelated diseases, I came to the realization four months ago that my general health was deteriorating rapidly even though I was only 30 years old. Only thirty, and already I had experienced:

- rheumatic fever, for 1 year

- chronic obesity-emaciation cycles, for 15 years

- hepatitis, for 1 year

- cystitis, on and off for 10 years

- crying spells, depression, and anxiety, for 3 years

- a complete physical and mental breakdown which forced me to abandon my work, 3 years ago

- episodes of excruciating back pain which recurred intermittently in three to five month intervals, for 10 years

Quite a terrifying list, I would say; and yet it took me fifteen years to conclude that I was in danger of becoming a cripple —permanently.

Sometimes it makes me wonder to look at my Ph.D. degree and to see, at the same time, the mist of personal neglect in which I was living. Although I had studied the subject extensively and had a fairly decent conception of how to eat properly and live a healthful life, I never applied what I knew to my day-to-day existence, even though I was extremely ill. I ate mostly protein and refined carbohydrates and I seldom got enough exercise.

And, what is more, it sometimes makes me absolutely shudder to consider the medical doctors with whom I have consulted, one after another, year after year, and to see how they have treated me. Rather than speaking of how to live healthfully, they have prescribed pain-killers and anti-biotics to suppress my symptoms.

But, four months ago, in desperation, I asked you for help and you gave it to me. You suggested, after hearing about my mysterious collection of chronic symptoms and diseases that I take a Glucose Tolerance Test. When I received the results, I found that, sure enough, I had a low blood sugar condition. After adhering to your diet for hypoglycemia for 3 months, I am feeling wonderful. My weight is stabilizing, my crying spells and depression have disappeared, I have had no backaches, and I have resumed my work. Not only did your diet correct my hypoglycemia, but it seems to be gradually correcting most of my other health problems as well.

The case of Mr. R. A., California

Dear Dr. Airola:

Six years ago I had a consultation with you in Los Angeles. You put me on your low-protein, high-natural-carbohydrate diet for hypoglycemia which, you said, you were testing at the time.

Last week, your friend, Dr. B. G., told me that you are writing a book on hypoglycemia, and I thought that you may wish to report on my case, since it is such a marvelous example of the nearly miraculous effect of your diet.

My history is probably in your files, but let me mention it briefly. I began feeling low blood sugar symptoms during my last year in high school. I could not concentrate on studies, I had constant headaches, and my mind seemed to be dull and confused. By the end of the school year, I was such a mental wreck that I failed finals, and, as a result, went on a destructive rampage and almost wrecked the school office building. I was arrested and kept in prison until my parents succeeded in getting me out on the basis of our family doctor's report that I was mentally sick. After two months in a mental hospital, I felt better and finally moved to California, enrolling in college. From the mid- 60's to the early 70's, my life was a veritable hell: drugs, alcohol, coffee, more drugs. Looking back at those years, I can't understand how I survived. Since my early high school years, and until I was 26, my nutrition consisted of practically nothing but ice cream, doughnuts, cokes, candies, potato chips, and an occasional hamburger. Yet, neither my family doctor, nor numerous doctors I have consulted with since, have ever asked questions about my diet.

Finally, a year before I saw you, I landed in prison for participating in disruptive activities; I then, again, moved to a mental hospital through the efforts of my parents. At the hospital, I was diagnosed schizophrenic. When I saw you, I was just released from the hospital and was still under heavy sedation. My parents brought me to you.

Today, I am totally healthy and a well-adjusted individual. My consultation with you has changed my life—in fact, it may have saved my life. You may remember that you requested a Glucose Tolerance Test. It showed a severe case of low blood sugar. You suggested I go to Dr. Buchinger's clinic in Germany, where my parents resided at the time. At Dr. Buchinger's clinic, I fasted on juices for twenty days. I felt like a clean, newborn baby after the fast, and all of my hypoglycemia symptoms disappeared. Then I went on Dr. Buchinger's diet for two months (his diet is practically identical with yours). Upon my return to the United States, I followed your diet strictly and am now taking all the vitamins and special supplements that you outlined for me. After only two years, I feel so healthy that now I can follow, more or less, the general lacto-vegetarian diet that you recommend in your books. I haven't had any symptoms of low blood sugar for the last three years. I am back in school now, completing my medical education, hoping eventually to be able to help others the way you helped me.

13

Recipes and Instructions

Special Hypoglycemia Drink

1 cup raw, whole, unpasteurized milk
  or: 1 cup kefir, yogurt, or other soured milk
  or: ½ cup fresh fruit juice and ½ cup water
½ small banana or equivalent of other fresh fruit
  (omit if fruit juice is used)
1 tsp. dry skim milk powder
1 tsp. brewer's yeast powder
1 tsp. flax seeds, sesame seeds, or chia seeds.

Place all ingredients in a blender and run on high until seeds are liquified. Drink slowly, or eat with a spoon.

Formula-H
Green Juice Cocktail

I have formulated this green juice specifically for hypoglycemics. It is extremely beneficial and healing, supplying valuable chlorophyl and an abundance of vitamins, minerals, trace elements, enzymes, coloring substances, and nature's own medicinal and healing factors. Jerusalem artichokes and avocado supply carbohydrates and sugars that are well tolerated by hypoglycemics without unfavorably affecting blood sugar levels.

Any available garden greens (parsley, lettuce, turnip tops, radish tops, wheat grass) or wild greens such as dandelions, common nettle, wild carrot tops, alfalfa, etc.
1 stalk celery
3-4 medium-size Jerusalem artichokes
¼ medium-size avocado

If you have an hydraulic-type juicer, all these ingredients can be ground and pressed together. If your juicer is an electric centrifugal juicer, which is the most common type, first make one glass of juice from celery and Jerusalem artichokes. Pour the juice into an electric *blender* and switch on low. Feed your greens and avocado into blender slowly. Finally, switch on high and liquify well. You may add kelp powder, and/or other natural herbs for flavoring, if you wish.

Drink slowly, salivating well. Best taken ½ hour to 1 hour before dinner. Two to three ounces is sufficient.

Homemade Applesauce

Any kind of apples may be used, but preferably organically grown sour apples such as Pippins, Roman Beauty, Jonathan, Northern Spy, Granny's, etc.

Wash apples well and remove stem. Cut into approximately 1-inch pieces. NOTE: Do not peel or remove core or seeds—use the whole apple. Place in a pan, and add one inch of water (only enough water to cover the bottom and prevent burning; glass, earthenware, or stainless steel utensils are best—*do not* use aluminum).

Cover, and bring to a boil. Simmer until apples are soft. Mash with potato masher, or place in a blender if finer texture is desired. Do not use sugar or honey, but pectin may be added if desired. When sauce is cooled, place in jars and refrigerate. Keeps for approximately one week.

Millet Cereal

1 cup hulled millet
3 cups water
½ tsp. honey
½ cup powdered skim milk

Rinse millet in warm water and drain. Place in a pan of water mixed with powdered skim milk and heat mixture to boiling point. Then simmer for ten minutes, stirring occasionally to prevent sticking and burning. Remove from heat and let stand for a half hour or more. Serve with milk, oil, or butter—or homemade applesauce. And treat yourself to the *most nutritious cereal in the world!*

Here's another, even better way to make millet cereal (or any other cereal, for that matter).

Place all ingredients in a pan with a tight cover. Use heatproof utensils: pyrex, earthenware or stainless steel, if possible. Put in an electric or gas oven turned to 200°, or less, and leave for 3–4 hours, or longer, if necessary; but the cereal will be ready to eat after about 3 hours. To speed the process, the cereal could be heated to boiling point before putting into the oven.

This cooking method is superior because of the low temperature, which makes the nutrients—especially the proteins—of millet or other grains more easily assimilable.

Kasha
(Buckwheat cereal)

1 cup whole buckwheat grains
2½ to 3 cups water

Bring water to a boil. Stir the buckwheat into the boiling water and let boil for two to three minutes. Turn heat to low and simmer for 15 to 20 minutes, stirring occasionally. If seasoning is desired use a very little sea salt. When all the water is absorbed, take from the stove and let stand for another 15 minutes. Kasha must never be mushy. Serve hot with sunflower seed oil, olive oil, sesame seed oil or butter. This is a favorite cereal in Russia and many other Eastern European countries. It has an unusual, mellow flavor and it is extremely nutritious. It contains complete proteins of high biological value, equal in quality to animal proteins as shown in recent studies.

Kasha can also be cooked the "oven way", as described above in the section on millet cereal.

I consider millet and buckwheat to be two of the most important cereals in the Hypoglycemic diet.

Buckwheat Pancakes

1 cup whole raw buckwheat
½ cup rolled oats or fresh wheat germ, which is not over 10 days old.
2 eggs
2 cups buttermilk, yogurt, or kefir
pinch of sea salt

Place whole buckwheat and oats in blender or seed grinder and grind well until a fine flour is obtained. Mix flour in a medium sized bowl with remaining ingredients and blend well. If batter is too thick, add fresh milk. Fry on a lightly buttered griddle on low heat.

Serve with butter, vegetable oil, or homemade applesauce. Makes 6 delicious medium-sized pancakes.

Waerland Five-Grain Kruska
(for four persons)

1 tbsp. whole wheat
1 tbsp. whole rye
1 tbsp. whole barley
1 tbsp. whole millet
1 tbsp. whole oats
2 tbsp. wheat bran

Take five grains and grind them coarsely in your grinder. Place in a pot with 1 to 1½ cups of water and add bran. Boil for 5 to 10 minutes, then wrap the pot in a blanket or news-papers and let it stand for a few hours. Experiment with the amount of water used—kruska must not be mushy, but should have the consistency of a very thick porridge. Serve hot with sweet milk and homemade applesauce, butter or vegetable oil.

Kruska is an extremely nutritious dish and should be eaten as a meal in itself.

Uncooked Quick Kruska

Use the same ingredients as above. Pour boiling water over the freshly ground grains and other ingredients and let stand and steep for half an hour. This quick *kruska* is delicious and more easily digested because of the preserved enzymes. Serve warm and eat the same way as the cooked *Five-Grain Kruska.*

How To Make Sprouts

First, make sure that the seeds or grains you buy for sprouting are packaged for food. Under no circumstances use seeds that are sold for planting; they more likely than not contain mercury compounds or other toxic chemicals. Play it safe and buy your seeds and sprouting grains at your health food store.

The seeds most commonly used for sprouting are: alfalfa, mung beans, soybeans and wheat.

There are many different methods of sprouting seeds. Slow germinating seeds, such as wheat or soybeans, can be soaked in water for two days (changing water twice a day) then spread thinly on a plate or paper towel for two or three days, rinsing them under running water three times a day to prevent molding.

Here's my own way of sprouting seeds: Place two table-spoons of alfalfa seeds in a quart size jar and fill with water. Let soak overnight. Rinse seeds well the following morning and return them to the glass jar without water, covering the jar with a cheese cloth held on by a rubber band. Keep rinsing the seeds three or four times a day. In two or three days, alfalfa sprouts are ready for eating. When seeds are fully sprouted, that is, the sprouts are one to two inches long, place the top on the jar and keep them in the refrigerator if they are not eaten right away. Always rinse sprouts before eating. Sprouts can be eaten as they are or mixed with salads or other foods. They can also be ground up in a drink, preferably with vegetable juices.

Homemade Yogurt

Take a bottle of skim milk and heat it almost to boiling, then cool to room temperature. Add two to three tablespoons of yogurt, which can be bought in a grocery store of health shop. Stir well. Pour into a wide-mouthed thermos bottle. Cover and let it stand overnight. In five to eight hours it will be solid and ready to serve. If you do not have a thermos jar, use an ordinary glass jar, and place it in a pan of warm water over an electric burner switched on "warm" for four to five hours, then switch off until milk is solid.

Use two to three spoonsful of your fresh, homemade yogurt as a culture for the next batch.

Homemade Kefir

To make your own kefir, you will need kefir grains. There is a mail order company, R.A. J. Biological Laboratory, 35 Park Ave., Blue Point, Long Island, New York, which sells kefir grains by mail directly to customers. The kefir grains will last indefinitely; there is never any need to reorder. Merely follow the instructions which will come with each order.

Place 1 tbsp. of kefir grains in a glass of milk, stir and allow to stand at room temperature overnight. When the milk coagulates, it is ready for eating. Strain and save the grains for the next batch. Kefir is a true "elixir of youth", used by centenarians in Bulgaria, Russia and Caucasus as an essential part of their daily diet.

Freeze-dried kefir culture, sold in health food stores, can also be used in making kefir.

Homemade Cottage Cheese (kvark)

Take homemade soured milk and warm it to about 110°F, by placing the container in warm water. When the milk has curdled, place a clean linen canvas or cheese cloth over a deep strainer and pour the curdled milk over it. Wait until all liquid whey has seeped through the strainer. What remains in the strainer is fresh, wholesome and delicious homemade cottage cheese. If the cheese is too hard, add a little sweet or sour cream, and stir. The higher the temperature, the harder the cheese, and vice versa. Raw homemade cottage cheese (kvark) can be made by straining soured milk through a fine cheese cloth, without warming it up first.

By the way, don't throw the whey away—it is an exceptionally nutritious and rejuvenating drink.

Homemade Soured Milk

Use only unpasteurized, raw milk. Place a bottle of milk in a pan filled with warm water, and warm it to about body temperature. Fill a cup or a deep plate, stir in a tablespoon of yogurt, cover with a paper towel (for dust) and keep in a warm place—for example, near the stove, radiator, or wherever there is a constant temperature. The milk will coagulate in approximately 24 hours.

Use one or two spoonfuls of soured milk as a culture for your next batch (use yogurt or commercial buttermilk only as a starting culture for the first batch).

Sour Rye Bread
(Black Bread Russian Style)

8 cups freshly ground whole rye flour
3 cups warm water
½ cup sourdough culture

Mix seven cups of flour with water and sourdough culture. Cover and let stand in a warm place for 12 to 18 hours. Add remaining flour and mix well. Place in greased pans. Let rise for approximately a half-hour. Bake at 350°F, one hour or more, if needed. Always save ½ cup of dough as a culture for the next baking. Keep the culture in a tightly closed jar in your refrigerator. For the initial baking it will be necessary to obtain a sourdough culture from a commercial baker.

This recipe makes 2 two-pound loaves.

Airola Salad

Here is a completely new variety of vegetable salad which I have specifically formulated for hypoglycemics. It can be, however, eaten with delight by anyone. It differs from the conventional vegetable salad in two distinctive ways:

1. It is "chunky"; it has no soft, leafy vegetables, such as lettuce, parsley, cabbage, spinach, or mustard greens.

2. It is "hot"; it has a distinct Mexican flavor, being spiced with chili (cayenne pepper), and lime or lemon.

Use the following fresh vegetables: avocados, carrots, tomatoes, green peppers, cucumbers, red onions, celery stalks, radish, and Jerusalem artichokes. If any of the above are not available, use what you can get. Tomatoes, cucumbers, green peppers, celery, and onions are the basic ingredients. Avocados and Jerusalem artichokes are of specific importance for hypoglycemics.

Chop all vegetables into about 1-inch pieces. Carrots can be sliced into ¼-inch thick slices. Do not peel cucumbers or Jerusalem artichokes.

Place all chopped vegetables in a bowl and add the following ingredients to taste: sea water or sea salt (available in health food stores), cayenne pepper or chili, paprika, lime or lemon juice. Add some water, stir briskly, and serve.

It is important to have lots of lime and lemon juice—at least the juice of ½ lime or ¼ lemon for each serving. That means, if you make a salad for four persons, use one lemon or two limes. It is best to eat the Airola salad with a spoon, being sure to consume all the dressing. This salad should be eaten as a meal in itself. Eat slowly and chew well. It is very filling and satisfying—and fantabulously delicious!

14

The Total Approach

In the last several years, a significant part of my time—
when I have not been writing or traveling around the world
doing research—has been spent in lecturing across the
United States and Canada, mostly on behalf of health-oriented organizations, to professional groups, universities,
and medical schools. Exposing one's ideas, especially those
that are new and contrary to orthodox thinking, to such a
huge number of listeners from vastly different backgrounds,
elicits a great number of varied responses: compliments,
praises, but also criticism, skepticism, and derision. One of
the most pleasing compliments, one that makes me feel my
work is worthwhile, and the one that I value most, is when I
am told that "I have it all together." In case you don't understand the modern vernacular of the new-age generation,
"having it all together" (in my specific field) means having
an understanding of the Concept of Totality when dealing
with various aspects of human life. "Having it all together"
means having a wholistic view of the problems of health and
disease as they relate to life and its purpose, as a whole.
"Having it all together" means the ability to see the entire
forest, not just a single tree; it means not losing view of the
human being as a complex, physical, mental, and spiritual
entity by undue emphasis on, or fascination with, a singular
aspect of his life.

Although most of my work—books, lectures, articles— deals with nutrition and how it is related to health and disease, I don't want to leave you with the impression that I have tunnel vision on the subject or that I consider nutrition to be the panacea and the only factor that is important for maintenance of health and prevention of disease. I speak and write of nutrition because I am primarily a nutritionist and a nutritionally-oriented naturopathic physician; therefore, nutrition is what you expect to learn from me. But I am fully aware of the fact that nutrition, as important a factor as it is in health and disease, is only *one* of several equally, if not more important, factors. These factors are: sufficient exercise; fresh air; sunshine; rest; relaxation; peace of mind; the absence of worries, tensions, and mental stresses; and, a positive outlook on life. To build and maintain optimum health, prevent disease, and live a long disease- and pain-free life, *all* these factors must be working together. This is what I call a *Total Approach to Health.*

The Concept of Biological Medicine

This principle of a Total Approach applies not only to maintenance of optimum health and prevention of disease, but also to *healing* of disease. According to the old Pasteurian concept of medicine, disease is caused by bacteria or virus which attack the unfortunate and undeserving individual who has no choice or responsibility for the fact that he becomes ill. (Does your doctor ask you what you eat or how you live when you see him for your health problems?) Orthodox medicine, which is still based on this outdated Pasteurian concept, believes that bacteria or germs are "going around", striking every unsuspecting person in their way. The job of a doctor is to kill or drive out the evil intruders with magic medicine power from injection needles or from miracle pills which will save the innocent victim from the vicious attack.

The new Biological Medicine takes exception to such a Pasteurian concept of disease and the symptomatic drug-therapy approach to the treatment of disease. The biological concept of medicine is based on the irrefutable physiological fact that the primary cause of disease is not the bacteria or virus, but *weakened resistance* brought about by man's own health-destroying living habits and physical and mental stresses. Thus, man must accept full responsibility for his own health.

Most diseases have the same basic underlying causes. These are the systemic derangement and the biochemical and metabolic disorders brought about by prolonged physical and mental stresses to which the individual has been subjected. Among these stress factors are: faulty nutritional patterns; systematic overeating; overindulgence in proteins, fats, or refined sugars; nutritional deficiencies; sluggish metabolism and consequent retention of toxic metabolic wastes; exogenous poisons from polluted food, water, air, and environment; toxic drugs; tobacco and alcohol; lack of sufficient exercise, rest and relaxation; and, severe physical and emotional stresses, tensions, worries, fears, etc. These health-destroying environmental factors bring about the derangement in the functions of all vital organs and glands with consequent biochemical imbalance in the tissues, auto-toxemia, chronic undersupply of oxygen to the cells, poor digestion and assimilation of nutrients, constipation . . . and *gradually lowered resistance to disease.* Thus, Biological Medicine considers not the bacteria, but the *weakened organism and the lowered resistance* to be the primary causes of disease. Bacteria is more often than not the *result* of disease, not its *cause.*

Since most conditions of ill health are systemic in their origin and have the same underlying causes, the basic treatment of all disease is likewise the same. First, all the underlying causes of disease must be eliminated—these causes are the health-destroying factors that produced ill health, including nutritional, physical, environmental, and emotional stresses and abuses. Second, the body's own healing, cleansing, and health-restoring activity must be supported by all means available, which include: optimum nutrition; specific vitamins and supplements; herbs and other effective natural medicines; supportive biological treatments such as hydrotherapy, cleansing fasts, massage, corrective exercises, rest, etc. If the patient is suffering from severe emotional stress and acute anxiety, his ability to absorb and utilize nutritional and medicinal factors is seriously impaired and effective healing will be prevented as long as emotional disturbances continue to act. Therefore, the patient must be given help that will enable him to free himself from all emotional stresses and worries and acquire a positive state of total relaxation and peace of mind.

Only such a *Total, Wholistic Approach* to healing can effect a complete restoration of health. It is not a matter of just treating and eliminating the symptoms of disease, but of treating the whole person by eliminating the underlying causes of his illness and helping the body to heal itself. This is the philosophy and the basic goal of Biological Medicine —the Medicine of the Future.

It is important that this concept of biological medicine and the Total Approach to health and healing be understood by hypoglycemics. By reading this and other books dealing with hypoglycemia, it is easy to get the impression that a dietary approach is all that is needed to restore health. I would have failed in my effort to create a useful, helpful manual on the effective treatment of hypoglycemia if I had not written a chapter to correct this false impression. A hypoglycemic—just as an arthritic, a diabetic, a heart patient, or any other sufferer of ill health—must fully realize that, as important as nutrition is, he cannot just eat his way to health. If the other important health-maintaining and healing factors are ignored, nutrition alone will fail to lead to optimum health. Only the total approach to healing can lead to total and complete restoration of optimum health.

Exercise

Life is motion. The most important nutrient that your body requires is not protein, vitamins, enzymes, fats, minerals . . . it is oxygen! You can live for years without any food, but for only five minutes without oxygen. Nutritionists, in their illustrative description of the body's mechanisms, like to compare it to an automobile. "Just as your car runs best on pure, high quality gas, so your body requires the highest quality food to run friction-free." This comparison is misleading. The automobile-gas relationship should be compared to the body-*oxygen* relationship. Oxygen is the most important nutrient that every organ and every cell of your body needs. How can you get enough of it?

Several times throughout this book I have referred to the effective and optimal functioning of your body as dependent on special bio-rhythms or life cycles, a kind of genetic programming which has been determined and formed as a result of man's adaptation to the historical and traditional circumstances of his environment. One of the environmental circumstances of prehistoric man was his great mobility connected with daily living. To survive, and provide nourishment, man had to move a great deal. And this he had to do on his own two legs. Much walking, running, moving about, and lifting was done during most of the day. Consequently, after thousands of years of adaptation to this kind of lifestyle, man's body was genetically programmed and adjusted to function efficiently on the level of oxygen that was generated by such a mobile life-style.

Now, our present life-style has eliminated 90 percent of the motion and exercise our bodies used to have. We do not move on our own power any more—cars, airplanes, and boats take care of that. We do not need to exercise our muscles to get our food—we simply drive to the super-market; and even there we use a cart to get food back to our car. Such a life-style results in a body which isn't getting much oxygen. The level of oxygen absorbtion is determined by the level of physical exertion. Our sedentary life has led to a chronic oxygen starvation. Our organs, muscles, brain, and nerves, which were designed to function at optimum capacity on a certain level of oxygen, now are forced to cope with their task on a constant undersupply of this most important nutrient. The consequences are obvious: physical and mental deterioration and a growing amount of disease that has developed since man has adopted his new, sedentary, mechanized environment, with its polluted air, where he is getting less and less oxygen.

How can you remedy this and give your body all the oxygen it needs to function efficiently and be disease-free? The only sensible solution is: *Get out in the fresh air and exercise!* I said "sensible" because, no doubt, man, with his ingenious and inventive mind, will soon discover less sensible ways to oxygenize his body, ways that will not require any effort on his own part, like taking oxygen pills or injections. Already, there are oxygen chambers and other gadgets where your body can be oxygenized. But, Mother Nature cannot be fooled. Your body is designed to function efficiently on optimum movement. Therefore, if you wish to obtain the optimum level of health and to prevent physical and mental deterioration, you must give it the movement it needs.

What exercises are best? Can yoga be sufficient? Can you get by with a few calisthenics in front of your TV each morning? Both yoga and TV calisthenics are good, but the exercise I am talking about, the kind that will help to saturate your whole body with oxygen, is a vigorous, exhausting, perspiration-causing activity such as jogging, running, playing tennis, swimming, or hard garden work—activity that will raise your heartbeat to 120–140 per minute.

Obviously, if you are totally inexperienced and un-trained, you shouldn't start your exercising by running five miles! Start by doing short, brisk morning walks and increase both time and speed gradually. Hypoglycemics, especially, must not over-exert in the beginning. Eventually, graduate to walking and jogging intermittently. If you have a garden (and if you don't, now is the time to start one right in your own back yard!), you can do a couple of hours work in the garden each morning. Don't give up yoga or bedroom cal-isthenics, but also take up tennis, or basketball, or swim-ming, or bike riding, or other vigorous exercises and/or games.

Remember: you simply *cannot* attain good health with-out plenty of exercise! You can eat the best food in the world, organic and all, take all the vitamins and supplements, read all the health books, and never miss a health lecture, but *if you do not exercise, regularly and vigorously, you will never enjoy good health.* Why do I say this so emphatically? Be-cause sufficient exercise is one of the irrefutable laws of health. And you cannot violate the laws of health and expect to escape paying a penalty in terms of ill health. For the benefit of those who go "into" nutrition so fanatically that they neglect all the other health-building and disease-pre-venting factors mentioned in this chapter, I dare to say:

"It is better to eat junk foods and exercise a lot, than to eat health foods and not exercise at all."

Now, there is a statement that will be surely mis-understood, misquoted, and misinterpreted. Please, re-read it carefully, and for the sake of your own health, make an effort to understand it. What I mean is that no amount of health food can make you healthy without sufficient ex-ercise. Without exercise, food cannot be properly digested and metabolized; it will only lead to poor assimilation, slug-gish elimination, constipation, auto-toxemia, and resultant disease and premature aging. But with plenty of vigorous exercise, even less perfect foods will be efficiently digested, nutrients well-utilized, elimination and body cleansing efficient, and health maintained. The *ideal,* of course, is to *eat health foods and exercise a lot!*

The medical evidence to the effect that ample regular exercise is imperative for optimum health is overwhelming. Exercise is absolutely essential to tone up your muscles, to improve digestion and metabolism, to maintain efficient nerve, lymph, and blood circulation, to prevent constipation, to assure the normal function of all organs and glands, and to supply enough oxygen to facilitate efficient cell and brain function. Keep in mind that the ultimate cause of all disease and premature aging is hypoxia, or lack of oxygen in your cells. The medical consensus is in complete agreement that our sedentary life contributes to many of our most dreaded diseases and is one of the main causes of one million yearly deaths from heart attacks in the United States!

Pure air, sun, rest, and relaxation

An Italian study showed that the prevalence of cancer was nine times greater among those who lived within 100 meters of moderately trafficked highways, as compared to those who lived further away. Think of all those who live in Los Angeles which is nothing but a solid network of busily trafficked freeways! It is well known that everyone over the age of twelve who lives in Los Angeles is affected by a certain degree of emphysema.

Pure, unpolluted air is getting more and more scarce. Yet, it is an absolute prerequisite to optimum health. If you live in a place where air is heavily polluted, you must make every effort to move to a place where you can breathe pure air. For the hypoglycemic, the access to pure air is of special importance. Most hypoglycemic symptoms are caused by oxygen starvation to the brain that results from low blood sugar level. Polluted, oxygen-poor air aggravates hypoglycemia. Carbon monoxide, the most dangerous substance in polluted air, interferes with oxygen utilization and causes hypoxia. If you wish to prevent hypoglycemia, or if you wish to correct your existing condition, continuous living in an area affected by smog will interfere with the accomplishment of your goals.

It is also imperative that you get an adequate amount of *sun*. Proper mineral metabolism is dependent on your body's being exposed to sun. Vitamin D is produced from the fatty particles on your skin when it is irradiated by the sun. Vitamin D is indispensable for many bodily functions, but especially for effective mineral utilization. Since vitamin D is very difficult to get from food, sufficient exposure to the sun is vital to health. Normal, healthy exposure is, however, different from over-exposure. Too much sun can be harmful, so do not overdo.

Rest and relaxation are other factors that must not be ignored. In this book, I have stressed repeatedly that stress is one of the main causes of disease. A certain amount of stress is natural, cannot be avoided, and is not harmful, if it is counteracted and balanced by sufficient rest and relaxation. Make a habit of having an afternoon nap or siesta. Relax with a good book or enjoyable music now and then. Don't drive yourself out of all energy reserves. Conserve energy and recharge your batteries by occasional pauses, breaks, and rest periods. This is of special value for hypoglycemics. Whatever you are occupied with, stop occasionally, take a short break, have a small snack, take a brisk walk. *Relax! Rest! Take it easy!*

Positive attitude and peace of mind

These are two other vital health factors that are missing in modern man's life. Emotional and mental stresses can tear your health down faster than inadequate nutrition can. It has been scientifically established that emotional and mental stresses—constant fears, anxieties, worries, tensions, depression, hate, jealousy, unhappiness, deprivation of love, and loneliness—can cause virtually every disease in the medical dictionary, including arthritis, ulcers, asthma, strokes, constipation, diabetes, high or low blood pressure, angina, glandular disturbances, sexual inadequacies, heart disease, hypoglycemia, and cancer.

The late J. I. Rodale, a brilliant medical and health writer, wrote once that "Happy people don't get cancer." Unbelievable as it may seem, this statement is fully substantiated by medical research. Happy people also don't get heart diseases or arthritis, or ulcers, or any other disease! A happy, peaceful, positive state of mind is the most powerful vaccination for the prevention of virtually any disease! And not for prevention only; for healing as well! A positive attitude, faith, belief in your body's own inherent power to heal itself, as well as reliance on the Greater Power for assistance, are the best medicines known to medical science.

Everyone has seen, heard, or read about miraculous healings performed by healers who use such unconventional modalities as the laying on of hands, holy waters, psychic surgery, or prayer. The implication is always that the healer possesses a great healing power. Actually, the great healing power that accomplishes such miraculous healing is within our own bodies; the healer merely helps to release it. Your body is equipped with the most powerful and the most effective healing system known to medical science. Your body is designed to be a self-cleansing, self-repairing, and self-healing mechanism. However, this healing power must be switched on by an act of faith before it can begin to work. Just as your room can be wired with electric power for brilliant light yet will remain in darkness until you switch the power on, so your own great healing capacity will remain untapped and unused, unless it is switched on by the act of faith. When Christ walked this earth and healed the sick, he used this same power to accomplish his miracles. Every time he was thanked for miraculous healing, he replied to the effect, Don't thank me—"thy faith made thee whole." Faith is not only the greatest healing power, but the greatest power known to man, period. This was realized by one of the greatest scientists and Nobel prize laureat, Prof. Alexis Carrel, who wrote in his classic book, MAN THE UNKNOWN, that "Prayer is the greatest power known to man." Prayer is an expression of faith. With faith *all* things are possible. Faith not only switches on the healing power within our body, but it releases all the vital energies that can potentiate any goal or accomplishment.

That a positive state of mind and the power of the subconscious can accomplish miraculous healings, was demonstrated on a large scale by the famous French physician, Dr. Emile Coué, in the beginning of this century. Dr. Coué achieved a world-wide reputation by curing thousands of people of every conceivable disease by a most unusual therapy. He sent patients back home, asking them to repeat aloud five times a day, the following words: "Every day, in every way, I am getting better, and better, and better!" To skeptics who laughed at such "nonsense", he said, "I don't care what you think, or even whether you believe it or not, just follow my prescription and you will be cured." And, sure enough, those who followed his advice saw to their amazement how every day, in every way, they did feel better, and better, and better; how their pains and ailments gradually disappeared; and how they eventually were totally cured! The loud repitition of the words had registered them on the subconscious mind, which "instructed" the healing powers within the body to initiate, and eventually to accomplish, the healing. The phenomenon of faith is actually a conviction on the subconscious, emotional level, as compared to mere belief, which is a conscious, intellectual process.

Relaxation, peace of mind, a positive outlook on life, a contented spirit, an absence of worries and fears, a cheerful disposition, unselfishness, love of mankind and faith in God —these are all powerful health-promoting factors without which optimum health cannot be achieved. And when health is lost, it cannot be restored *unless* the adequate nutritional and biological therapeutic program is "supplemented" with a good dose of "vitamin X": peace of mind, positive attitude, happy disposition, and faith in God—the faith that Nature and God will do *their parts* in helping to restore health, if we do *our part.*

Why better health?

Moreover, the motivation for the attainment of better health must be right. The real purpose of attaining better physical health and longer life is not just the mere enjoyment of a pain- and disease-free existence, but a higher, divine purpose for which life was given to us. All endeavors toward attaining better health would be wasted efforts unless the healthy body is used as a worthy temple in which the spirit will dwell and be developed. The purpose of our lives is not just the building of magnificent biceps and beautiful bodies, but perfecting and refining our divine spirit and becoming more God-like. "Be ye perfect, even as your Father, which is in heaven, is perfect", said the Master from Nazareth. Our life on this planet at this time in history, is just a short episode in the eternal divine plan of human development and progression—a schooling period aimed at improving and perfecting our human and divine characteristics.

Although this book deals mostly with nutritional and other physical aspects of preventing disease and restoring health, I wish to emphasize that there is a divine nature and purpose to all life, and that the real reason for achieving good health and building a strong, healthy body, is to prepare a way for our spiritual growth and perfection. Freed from disease and pain, we can pursue our true purpose in life—the perfection and refinement of our divine spirit. Only when our efforts to improve physical health are thus motivated will they fit into the framework of the purposeful, divinely-designed plan for our lives.

RECOMMENDED DAILY

(Designed for the maintenance of good nutrition

BASED ON TABLES PUBLISHED BY FOOD AND NUTRITION RESEARCH COUNCIL.

	AGE From up to years	WEIGHT		HEIGHT		ENERGY CALORIES	PROTEIN	FAT-SOLUBLE VITAMINS		
								VITAMIN A ACTIVITY	VITAMIN D	VITAMIN E ACTIVITY
		kg.	lb.	cm.	in.	KCAL	GM	I.U.	I.U.	I.U.
INFANTS	0.0-0.5	6	14	60	24	kg. x 117	kg. x 2.2	1,400	400	4
	0.5-1.0	9	20	71	28	kg. x 108	kg. x 2.0	2,000	400	5
CHILDREN	1-3	13	28	86	34	1,300	23	2,000	400	7
	4-6	20	44	110	44	1,800	30	2,500	400	9
	7-10	30	66	135	54	2,400	36	3,300	400	10
MALES	11-14	44	97	158	63	2,800	44	5,000	400	12
	15-18	61	134	172	69	3,000	54	5,000	400	15
	19-22	67	147	172	69	3,000	52	5,000	400	15
	23-50	70	154	172	69	2,700	56	5,000	–	15
	51+	70	154	172	69	2,400	56	5,000	–	15
FEMALES	11-14	44	97	155	62	2,400	44	4,000	400	10
	15-18	54	119	162	65	2,100	48	4,000	400	11
	19-22	58	128	162	65	2,100	46	4,000	400	12
	23-50	58	128	162	65	2,000	46	4,000	–	12
	51+	58	128	162	65	1,800	46	4,000	–	12
	Pregnant					+300	+30	5,000	400	15
	Lactating					+500	+20	6,000	400	15

DIETARY ALLOWANCES

of practically all healthy people in the U.S.A.)

BOARD, NATIONAL ACADEMY OF SCIENCE, NATIONAL
Revised 1973

	WATER-SOLUBLE VITAMINS						MINERALS					
VITAMIN C	FOLACIN	NIACIN	B_2	B_1	B_6	B_{12}	CALCIUM	PHOSPHORUS	IODINE	IRON	MAGNESIUM	ZINC
mg	mcg.	mg.	mg.	mg.	mg.	mcg.	mg.	mg.	mcg.	mg.	mg.	mg.
35	50	5	0.4	0.3	0.3	0.3	360	240	35	10	60	3
35	50	8	0.6	0.5	0.4	0.3	540	400	45	15	70	5
40	100	9	0.8	0.7	0.6	1.0	800	800	60	15	150	10
40	200	12	1.1	0.9	0.9	1.5	800	800	80	10	200	10
40	300	16	1.2	1.2	1.2	2.0	800	800	100	10	250	10
45	400	18	1.5	1.4	1.6	3.0	1,200	1,200	130	18	350	15
45	400	20	1.8	1.5	1.8	3.0	1,200	1,200	150	18	400	15
45	400	20	1.8	1.5	2.0	3.0	800	800	140	10	350	15
45	400	18	1.6	1.4	2.0	3.0	800	800	130	10	350	15
45	400	16	1.5	1.2	2.0	3.0	800	800	110	10	350	15
45	400	16	1.3	1.2	1.6	3.0	1,200	1,200	115	18	300	15
45	400	14	1.4	1.1	2.0	3.0	1,200	1,200	115	18	300	15
45	400	14	1.4	1.1	2.0	3.0	800	800	100	18	300	15
45	400	13	1.2	1.0	2.0	3.0	800	800	100	18	300	15
45	400	12	1.1	1.0	2.0	3.0	800	800	80	10	300	15
60	800	+2	+0.3	+0.3	2.5	4.0	1,200	1,200	125	18+	450	20
60	600	+4	+0.5	+0.3	2.5	4.0	1,200	1,200	150	18	450	25

COMPOSITION OF FOODS
100 grams, edible portion

(dash (—) denotes lack of reliable data for a constituent believed to be present in measurable amount)

FOOD	CALORIES	PROTEINS grams	FATS grams	CARBOHYDRATES grams	CALCIUM mg.	PHOSPHORUS mg.	MAGNESIUM mg.	IRON mg.	SODIUM mg.	POTASSIUM mg.	VITAMIN A VALUE IU	B₁ mg.	B₂ mg.	NIACIN mg.	VITAMIN C mg.
ACEROLA cherry, raw	28	.4	.3	6.8	12	11	—	.2	8	83	—	.02	.06	0.4	1,300
ACEROLA JUICE, raw	23	.4	.3	4.8	10	9	—	.5	3	—	—	.02	.06	.4	1,600
ALMONDS, dried	598	18.6	54.2	19.5	234	504	270	4.7	4	773	0	.24	.92	3.5	trace
APPLES, freshly harvested	58	.2	.6	14.5	7	10	8	.3	1	110	90	.03	.02	.4	7-20
APPLE JUICE, canned or bottled	47	.1	trace	11.9	6	9	4	.6	1	101	—	.01	.02	.1	1
APRICOTS, raw	51	1.0	.2	12.8	17	23	12	.5	1	281	2,700	0.3	.04	.6	10
APRICOTS, dried, uncooked	260	5.0	.5	66.5	67	108	62	5.5	26	979	10,900	.01	.16	3.3	12
ARTICHOKES, globe or French, raw	9-47	2.9	0.2	10.6	51	88	—	1.3	43	430	160	.08	.05	1.0	12
cooked	8-44	2.8	.2	9.6	51	68	—	1.1	30	301	150	.07	.04	.7	8
ARTICHOKES, Jerusalem, raw	7-75	2.3	.1	16.7	14	78	11	3.4	—	—	20	.2	.06	1.3	4
ASPARAGUS, raw spears	26	2.5	.2	5.0	22	62	20	1.0	2	278	900	.18	.20	1.5	33
cooked spears	20	2.2	.2	3.6	21	50	14	.6	1⁺	183	900	.16	.18	1.4	26
AVOCADOS, raw	167	2.1	16.4	6.3	10	42	45	.6	4	604	290	.11	.20	1.6	14
BANANAS, common, raw	85	1.1	.2	22.2	8	26	33	.7	1	370	190	.05	.06	.7	10
BARLEY, pearled, light	349	8.2	1.0	78.8	16	189	37	2.0	3	160	0	.12	.05	3.1	0

BEANS, common white, cooked	118	7.8	.6	21.2	50	148	37	2.7	7	416	0	.14	.07	.7	0
red, cooked	347	7.8	.5	21.4	38	140	—	2.7	3	340	trace	.11	.06	.7	—
pinto, raw	349	22.9	1.2	63.7	135	457	46	6.4	10	984	—	.84	.21	2.2	—
lima, immature cooked	123	8.4	.5	22.1	52	142	48	2.8	2	650	290	.24	.12	1.4	29
lima, mature, cooked	138	8.2	.6	25.6	29	154	—	3.1	2	612	—	.13	.06	.7	—
mung, sprouted, raw	38	3.8	.2	6.6	19	64	32	1.3	5	223	20	.13	.13	.8	19
green, raw	32	1.9	.2	7.1	56	44	21	.8	7	243	600	.08	.11	.5	19
green, cooked	25	1.6	.2	5.4	50	37	25	.6	4	151	540	.07	.09	.5	12
BEETS, red, raw	43	1.6	.1	9.9	16	33	15	.7	60	335	20	.03	.05	.4	10
red, cooked	32	1.1	.1	7.2	14	23	—	.5	43	208	20	.03	.04	.3	6
BEET GREENS, raw	24	2.2	.3	4.6	119	40	106	3.3	130	570	6,100	.10	.22	.4	30
cooked	18	1.7	.3	3.3	99	25	—	1.9	76	332	5,000	.07	.15	.3	15
BLACKBERRIES, raw	58	1.2	.9	12.9	32	19	30	.9	1	170	200	.03	.04	.4	21
BLUEBERRIES, raw	62	.7	.5	15.3	15	13	6	1.0	—	81	100	.03	.06	.5	14
BRAZIL NUTS, raw	654	14.3	66.9	10.9	186	693	225	3.4	1	715	trace	.96	.12	1.6	—
BROCCOLI, raw spears	32	3.6	.3	5.9	103	78	24	1.1	15	382	2,500	.10	.23	.9	113
cooked	26	3.1	.3	4.5	88	62	21	.8	10	267	2,500	.09	.20	.8	90
BRUSSELS SPROUTS, raw	45	4.9	.4	8.3	36	80	29	1.5	14	390	550	.10	.16	.9	102
cooked	36	4.2	.4	6.4	32	72	21	1.1	10	273	520	.08	.14	.8	87
BUCKWHEAT, whole grain	335	11.7	2.4	72.9	114	282	229	3.1	—	448	0	.60	—	4.4	0
BUTTER, salted	716	.6	81.	.4	20	16	2	0	987	23	3,300	—	—	—	0
unsalted	720	.6	82.	.4	20	16	—	0	8	9	3,350	—	—	0	—
BUTTERMILK, cultured, from skim milk	36	3.6	.1	5.1	121	95	14	trace	130	140	trace	.04	.18	.1	1
CABBAGE, white, raw	24	1.3	.2	5.4	49	29	13	.4	20	233	130	.05	.05	.3	47
red, raw	31	2.0	.2	6.9	42	35	—	.8	26	268	40	.09	.06	.4	61
savoy, raw	24	2.4	.2	4.6	67	54	—	.9	22	269	200	.05	.08	.3	55
CAROB FLOUR	180	4.5	1.4	80.7	352	81	23	—	—		—	—	—	—	—
CARROTS, raw	42	1.1	.2	9.7	37	36	—	.7	47	341	11,000	.06	.05	.6	8
CASHEW NUTS	561	17.2	45.7	29.3	38	373	267	3.8	15	464	100	.43	.25	1.8	—
CAULIFLOWER, raw	27	2.7	.2	5.2	25	56	24	1.1	13	295	60	.11	.10	.7	78
cooked	22	2.3	.2	4.1	21	42	—	.7	9	206	60	.09	.08	.6	55
CELERY, raw	17	.9	.1	3.9	39	28	22	.3	126	341	240	.03	.03	.3	9
CHARD, Swiss, raw	25	2.4	.3	4.6	88	39	65	3.2	147	550	6,500	.06	.17	.5	32
cooked	18	1.8	.2	3.3	73	24	—	1.8	86	321	5,400	.04	.11	.4	16

FOOD	CALORIES	PROTEINS grams	FATS grams	CARBOHYDRATES grams	CALCIUM mg.	PHOSPHORUS mg.	MAGNESIUM mg.	IRON mg.	SODIUM mg.	POTASSIUM mg.	VITAMIN A VALUE IU	B1 mg.	B2 mg.	NIACIN mg.	VITAMIN C mg.
CHEESE, Blue or Roquefort	368	21.5	30.5	2.0	315	339	48	.5	700	82	1,240	.03	.61	1.2	
Cheddar	398	25.0	32.2	2.1	750	478	45	1.0	229	85	1,310	.03	.46	.1	
Cottage, creamed	106	13.6	4.2	2.9	94	152	—	.3	290	72	170	.03	.25	.1	
Cottage, uncreamed	86	17.0	.3	2.7	90	175	—	.4	710	104	10	.03	.28	.1	
Swiss	370	27.5	28.0	1.7	925	563	—	.9			1,140	.01	.40	.1	
Brick	370	22.2	30.5	1.9	730	455	—	.9			1,240	—	.45	.1	
CHERRIES, sour, red, raw	58	1.2	.3	14.3	29	19	14	.4	2	191	1,000	.05	.06	.4	10
sweet, raw	70	1.3	.3	17.4	22	19	9	.4	2	191	110	.05	.06	.4	10
frozen, sour, red	55	1.0	.4	13.4	13	22	10	.7	2	188	1,000	.04	.07	.3	5
CHESTNUTS, fresh	194	2.9	1.5	42.1	27	88	41	1.7	6	454	—	.22	.22	.6	—
COCONUT MEAT, fresh	346	3.5	35.3	9.4	13	95	46	1.7	23	256	0	.05	.02	.5	3
dried	662	7.2	64.9	23.0	26	187	90	3.3	—	588	0	.06	.04	.6	0
COCONUT WATER, from green coconuts	22	.3	.2	4.7	20	13	28	.3	25	147	0	trace	trace	.1	2
COLLARDS, raw, leaves	45	4.8	.8	7.5	250	82	57	1.5	—	450	9,300	0.16	.31	1.7	152
cooked	33	3.6	.7	5.1	188	52	38	.8	—	262	7,800	.11	.20	1.2	76
CORN, whole-grain, dried, raw	348	8.9	3.9	72.0	22	268	147	2.1	1	284	490	.37	.12	2.2	—
SWEET, on-the-cob, raw	96	3.5	1.0	22.0	3	111	48	.7	trace	280	400	.15	.12	1.7	12
cooked on the cob	91	3.3	1.0	21.0	3	89	19	.6	trace	196	400	.12	.10	1.4	9
flour	368	7.8	2.6	76.8	6	164	106	1.8	1	—	340	.20	.06	1.4	—
bread, whole-grain	207	7.4	7.2	29.1	120	211	—	1.1	628	157	150	.13	.19	.6	1
CRANBERRIES, raw	46	.4	.7	10.8	14	10	8	.5	2	82	40	.03	.02	.1	11
CUCUMBERS, raw	15	.9	.1	3.4	25	27	11	1.1	6	160	250	.03	.04	.2	11

Food	Calories	Protein	Fat	Carbohydrate	Calcium	Phosphorus	Magnesium	Iron	Sodium	Potassium	Vitamin A	Thiamine	Riboflavin	Niacin	Ascorbic Acid
CURRANTS, black, raw	54	1.7	.1	13.1	60	40	15	1.1	3	372	230	.05	.05	.3	200
DANDELION GREENS, raw	45	2.7	.7	9.2	187	66	36	3.1	76	397	14,000	.19	.26		35
DATES	274	2.2	.5	72.9	59	63	58	3.0	1	648	50	.09	.10	2.2	0
EGGS, whole, raw	163	12.9	11.5	.9	54	205	11	2.3	122	129	1,180	.11	.30	.1	0
yolks, raw	348	16.0	30.6	.6	141	569	16	5.5	52	98	3,400	.22	.44	.1	0
cooked, whole	163	12.9	11.5	.9	54	205		2.3	122	129	1,180	.09	.28	.1	0
EGGPLANT, cooked	19	1.0	.2	4.1	11	21		.6		150	10	.05	.04	.5	3
ELDERBERRIES, raw	72	2.6	.5	16.4	38	28	10	1.6	14	300	600	.07	.06	.5	36
ENDIVE, raw	20	1.7	.1	4.1	81	54	20	1.7	2	294	3,300	.07	.14	.5	10
FIGS, raw	80	1.2	.3	20.3	35	22		.6	2	194	80	.06	.05	.4	2
dried	274	4.3	1.3	69.1	126	77	71	3.0	34	640	80	.10	.10	.7	0
FILBERTS (hazelnuts)	634	12.6	62.4	16.7	209	337	184	3.4	2	704		.46		.9	trace
GARLIC, raw	137	6.2	.2	30.8	29	202	36	1.5	19	529	trace	.25	.08	.5	15
GOOSEBERRIES, raw	39	0.8	.2	9.7	18	15	9	0.5	1	155	290				33
GRAPEFRUIT, raw	41	.5	.1	10.6	16	16	12	.4	1	135	80	.04	.02	.2	38
juice	39	.5	.1	9.2	9	15	12	.2	1	162	80	.04	.02	.2	38
GRAPES, raw	69	1.3	1.0	15.7	16	12	13	.4	3	158	100	.05	.03	.3	4
juice, bottled	66	.2	trace	16.6	11	12	13	.3	2	116		.04	.02	.2	trace
GUAVAS, whole, raw	62	.8	.6	15.	23	42	13	.9	4	289	280	.05	.05	1.2	242
HONEY	304	.3	0	82.3	5	6	3	.5	5	51	0	trace	.04	.3	1
HORSERADISH, raw	87	3.2	.3	19.7	140	64	34	1.4	8	564		.07			81
KALE, leaves, raw	53	6.0	.8	9.0	249	93	37	2.7	75	378	10,000	.17	.26	2.1	186
cooked	39	4.5	.7	6.1	187	58		1.6	43	221	8,300	.10	.18	1.6	93
KELP, raw		5.0	1.1		1,093	240	740	3.7	3,007	5,273					5-140
KOHLRABI, raw	29	2.0	.1	6.6	41	51	37	.5	8	372	20	.06	.04	.3	66
KUMQUATS, raw	65	.9	.1	17.1	63	23		.4	7	236	600	.08	.10		36
LEMONS, peeled, raw	27	1.1	.3	8.2	26	16	10	.6	2	138	20	.04	.02	.1	53
LEMON JUICE, raw	25	.5	.2	8.0	7	10	8	.2	1	141	20	.03	.01	.1	46
LENTILS, dry, cooked	106	7.8	trace	19.3	25	119	80	2.1		249	20	.07	.06	.6	0
LETTUCE, raw, romaine	18	1.3	.3	3.5	68	25		1.4	9	264	1,900	.05	.08	.4	18
Iceberg, New York	13	.9	.1	2.9	20	22	11	.5	9	175	330	.06	.06	.3	6
MANGOS, raw	66	.7	.4	16.8	10	13	18	.4	7	189	4,800	.05	.05	1.1	35

FOOD	CALORIES	PROTEINS grams	FATS grams	CARBOHYDRATES grams	CALCIUM mg.	PHOSPHORUS mg.	MAGNESIUM mg.	IRON mg.	SODIUM mg.	POTASSIUM mg.	VITAMIN A VALUE IU	B₁ mg.	B₂ mg.	NIACIN mg.	VITAMIN C mg.
MILK, cow's, whole	65	3.5	3.5	4.9	118	93	13	trace	50	144	140	.03	.17	.1	1
skim	36	3.6	.1	5.1	121	95	14	trace	52	145	trace	.04	.18	.1	1
dry, whole	502	26.4	27.5	38.2	909	708	98	.5	405	1,330	1,130	.29	1.46	.7	6
dry, skim non-instant	363	35.9	.8	52.3	1,308	1,016	143	.6	532	1,745	30	.35	1.80	.9	7
MILK, goat's, raw	67	3.2	4.0	4.6	129	106	17	.1	34	180	160	.04	.11	.3	1
MILLET, whole-grain	327	9.9	2.9	72.9	20	311	162	6.8	—	430	0	.73	.38	2.3	0
MOLASSES, blackstrap	213	—	—	55	684	84	258	16.1	96	2,927	—	.11	.19	2.0	—
MUSHROOMS, cultivated, raw	28	2.7	.3	4.4	6	116	13	.8	15	414	trace	.10	.46	4.2	3
MUSKMELONS, raw, cantaloupe	30	.7	.1	7.5	14	16	16	.4	12	251	3,400	.04	.03	.6	33
honeydew	33	.8	.3	7.7	14	16	16	.4	12	251	40	.04	.03	.6	23
MUSTARD GREENS, raw	31	3.0	.5	5.6	183	50	27	3.0	32	377	7,000	.11	.22	.8	97
NECTARINES, raw	64	.6	trace	17.1	4	24	13	.5	6	294	1,650	—	—	—	13
OATMEAL or rolled oats, dry cooked	390	14.2	7.2	68.2	53	405	144	4.5	2	352	0	.60	.14	1.0	0
OKRA, raw	55	2.0	1.0	9.7	9	57	21	.6	—	61	0	.08	.02	.1	0
ONIONS, mature, raw	36	2.4	.3	7.6	92	51	41	.6	3	249	520	.17	.21	1.0	31
green, bulb & top	36	1.5	.1	8.7	27	36	12	.5	10	157	40	.03	.04	.2	10
ORANGES, peeled, raw	49	1.5	.2	8.2	51	39	—	1.0	5	237	2,000	.05	.05	.4	32
ORANGE JUICE, raw	45	1.0	.2	12.2	41	20	11	.4	1	200	200	.10	.04	.4	50
PAPAYA, raw	39	.7	.1	10.2	11	17	11	.3	3	200	200	.09	.03	.3	50
PARSLEY, raw	44	3.6	.6	10.0	20	16	41	6.2	45	234	1,750	.04	.04	.3	56
PARSNIPS, raw	76	1.7	.5	8.5	203	63	32	.7	12	727	8,500	.12	.26	1.2	56
PEACHES, raw	38	.6	.1	17.5	50	77	10	.5	1	541	30	.07	.08	.1	10
PEANUTS, raw, with skins	564	26.0	47.5	18.6	69	401	206	2.1	5	674	—	1.14	.13	17.2	0

PEARS, raw	61	.7	.4	15.3	8	11	7	.3	2	130	20	.02	.04	.1	4
PEAS, raw, from pods	53	3.4	.2	12.0	62	90	35	.7	—	170	680	.28	.12	—	21
green, cooked	71	5.4	.4	12.1	23	99	—	1.8	1	196	540	.28	.11	2.3	20
split, cooked	115	8.0	.3	20.8	11	89	—	1.7	13	296	40	.15	.09	.9	—
PECANS	687	9.2	71.2	14.6	73	289	142	2.4	trace	603	130	.86	.13	.9	2
PEPPERS, raw, sweet, green	22	1.2	.2	4.8	9	22	18	.7	13	213	420	.08	.08	.5	128
raw, red	31	1.4	.3	7.1	13	30	—	.6	—	—	4,450	.08	.08	.5	204
PERSIMMONS, raw	127	.8	.4	33.5	27	26	8	2.5	1	310	—	—	—	—	66
PINEAPPLE, raw	52	.4	0.2	13.7	17	8	13	0.5	1	146	70	.09	.03	.2	17
juice, canned, unsweetened	55	.4	.2	13.5	15	9	12	.3	1	149	50	.05	.02	.2	9
PLUMS, prune-type, raw	75	.8	.2	19.7	12	18	9	.5	1	170	300	.03	.03	.5	4
POTATOES, raw	76	2.1	.1	17.1	7	53	34	.6	3	407	trace	.10	.04	1.5	20
baked in skin	93	2.6	.1	21.1	9	65	—	.7	4	503	trace	.10	.04	1.7	20
boiled in skin	76	2.1	.1	17.1	7	53	—	.6	3	407	trace	.09	.04	1.5	16
PUMPKIN, raw	26	1.0	.1	6.5	21	44	12	.8	1	340	1,600	.05	.11	.6	9
PUMPKIN SEEDS, dry	553	29.0	46.7	15.0	51	1,144	—	11.2	—	—	70	.24	.19	2.4	—
RADISHES, raw	17	1.0	.2	3.6	30	31	15	1.0	18	322	10	.03	.03	.3	26
RAISINS, natural, uncooked	289	2.5	.2	77.4	62	101	35	3.5	27	763	20	.11	.08	.5	1
RASPBERRIES, raw, black	73	1.5	1.4	15.7	30	22	30	0.9	1	199	trace	.03	.09	.9	18
red	57	1.2	.5	13.6	22	22	20	0.9	1	168	130	.03	.09	.9	25
RICE, brown, cooked	119	2.5	.6	25.5	12	73	29	.5	3	70	0	.09	.02	1.4	0
RICE BRAN	276	13.3	15.8	50.8	76	1,386	—	19.4	trace	1,495	0	2.26	.25	29.8	0
RICE POLISHINGS	265	12.1	12.8	57.7	69	1,106	—	16.1	trace	714	0	1.84	.18	28.2	0
RUTABAGAS, raw	46	1.1	.1	11.0	66	39	15	.4	5	239	580	.07	.07	1.1	43
cooked	35	.9	.1	8.2	59	31	—	.3	4	167	550	.06	.06	.8	26
RYE, whole-grain	334	12.1	1.7	73.4	38	376	115	3.7	1	467	0	.43	.22	1.6	0
flour, dark	327	16.3	2.6	68.1	54	536	73	4.5	1	860	0	.61	.22	2.7	0
SAUERKRAUT, solids and liquid	18	1.0	.2	4.0	36	18	—	.5	—	140	50	.03	.04	.2	14
SESAME SEEDS, dry, whole	563	18.6	49.1	21.6	1,160	616	181	10.5	60	725	30	.98	.24	5.4	0
SOYBEANS, dry, raw	403	34.1	17.7	33.5	226	554	265	8.4	5	1,677	80	1.10	.31	2.2	—
cooked	130	11.0	5.7	10.8	73	179	—	2.7	2	540	30	.21	.09	.6	0
sprouted, raw	46	6.2	1.4	5.3	48	67	—	1.0	—	—	80	.23	.20	.8	13
sprouted, cooked	38	5.3	1.4	3.7	43	50	—	.7	—	—	80	.16	.15	.7	4

SOYBEAN CURD (TOFU)	72	7.8	4.2	2.4	128	126	111	1.9	7	42	0	.06	.03	.1	—
SOYBEAN FLOUR, full-fat	421	36.7	20.3	30.4	199	558	247	8.4	1	1,660	110	.85	.31	2.1	0
SOYBEAN MILK, powder	429	41.8	20.3	28.0	278	—	300	—	—	—	—	—	—	—	—
SPINACH, raw	26	3.2	.3	4.3	93	51	88	3.1	71	470	8,100	.10	.20	.6	51
cooked	23	3.0	.3	3.6	93	38	65	2.2	50	324	8,000	.07	.14	.5	28
SQUASH, summer, all varieties, raw	19	1.1	.1	4.2	28	29	16	.4	1	202	410	.05	.09	1.0	22
cooked	14	.9	.1	3.1	25	25	16	.4	1	141	370	.05	.08	.8	10
winter, raw	50	1.4	.3	12.4	22	38	17	.6	1	369	3,700	.05	.11	.6	13
cooked (baked)	63	1.8	.4	15.4	28	48	17	.8	1	461	4,200	.05	.13	.7	13
STRAWBERRIES, raw	37	.7	.5	8.4	21	21	12	1.0	1	164	60	.03	.07	.6	59
SUNFLOWER SEED KERNELS, dry	560	24.0	47.3	19.9	120	837	38	7.1	30	920	50	1.96	.23	5.4	—
TOMATOES, ripe, raw	22	1.1	.2	4.7	13	27	14	.5	3	244	900	.06	.04	.7	23
TOMATO JUICE, canned	19	.9	.1	4.3	7	18	10	.9	200	227	800	.05	.03	.8	16
TURNIPS, raw	30	1.0	.2	6.6	39	30	20	.5	49	268	trace	.04	.07	.6	36
cooked	23	.8	.2	4.9	35	24	—	.4	34	188	trace	.04	.05	.3	22
TURNIP GREENS, raw	28	3.0	.3	5.0	246	58	58	1.8	—	—	7,600	.21	.39	.8	139
WALNUTS, black	628	20.5	59.3	14.8	trace	570	190	6.0	3	460	300	.22	.11	.7	—
English	651	14.8	64.0	15.8	99	380	131	3.1	2	450	30	.33	.13	.9	2
WATERCRESS, raw	19	2.2	.3	3.0	151	54	20	1.7	52	282	4,900	.08	.16	.9	79
WATERMELON, raw	26	.5	.2	6.4	7	10	8	.5	1	100	590	.03	.03	.2	7
WHEAT, whole-grain, spring	330	14.0	2.2	69.1	36	383	160	3.1	3	370	—	.57	.12	4.3	0
winter	330	12.3	1.8	71.7	46	354	160	3.4	3	370	—	.52	.12	4.3	0
WHEAT BRAN	213	16.0	4.6	61.9	119	1,276	490	14.9	9	1,121	0	.72	.35	21.0	0
WHEAT GERM, raw	363	26.6	10.9	46.7	72	1,118	336	9.4	3	827	0	2.01	.68	4.2	0
WHEY, powder	349	12.9	1.1	73.5	646	589	130	1.4	—	—	50	.50	2.51	.8	0
YAM, tuber, raw	101	2.1	.2	23.2	20	69	31	.6	—	600	trace	.10	.04	.5	9
YEAST, brewer's debittered	283	38.8	1.0	38.4	210	1,753	231	17.3	121	1,894	trace	15.61	4.28	37.9	trace
torula	277	38.6	1.0	37.0	424	1,713	165	19.3	15	2,046	trace	14.01	5.06	44.4	trace
YOGURT, from whole milk	62	3.0	3.4	4.9	111	87	12	trace	47	132	140	.03	.16	.1	1
from skimmed milk	50	3.4	1.7	5.2	120	94	13	trace	51	143	70	.04	.18	.1	1

SOURCES: Agriculture Handbook No. 8., U.S. Dept. Agric. Washington, D.C.; Home and Garden Bulletin No. 72.

REFERENCES

1. Adams, Ruth and Murray, Frank, *Is Low Blood Sugar Making You a Nutritional Cripple?*, Introduction by Robert C. Atkins, M.D., P.C., Larchmont Books, N.Y., N.Y., 1975, p. 5.
2. Cheraskin, E., Ringsdorf, W. M., and Brecher, Arline, *Psychodietetics: Food as the Key to Emotional Health*, Stein and Day, N.Y., N.Y., 1974.
3. Ross, Harvey M., *The Journal of Orthomolecular Psychiatry*, Vol. 3, No. 4.
4. Fredericks, Carlton, "Hotline," *Prevention*, July, 1975, p. 51.
5. Rodale, J. I., *Encyclopedia of Common Diseases*, Rodale Press, Emmaus, Pa., 1970.
6. Airola, Paavo, *How to Keep Slim, Healthy, and Young With Juice Fasting*, Health Plus Publishers, P.O. Box 22001, Phoenix, AZ., 1971.
7. Fredericks, Carlton, and Goodman, Herman, *Low Blood Sugar and You*, Grosset & Dunlap, N.Y., 1969.
8. Tintera, John W., *Journal of the American Geriatric Society*, February, 1966.
9. Airola, Paavo, *How To Get Well*, Health Plus Publishers, P.O. Box 22001, Phoenix, AZ., 1974.
10. Gyland, Dr. Stephen, from his letter to the *Journal of the American Medical Association*, Vol. 152, July 18, 1953.
11. Harris, Seale, the *Journal of the American Medical Association*, 1924.
12. Adrenal Metabolic Research Society of Hypoglycemia Foundation, Inc., P.O. Box 98, Fleetwood, Mount Vernon, N.Y., 10552.
13. Salzer, Harry M., from papers delivered before the Section of Nervous and Mental Diseases at the meeting of the American Medical Association, August, 1965, as reported by Dr. Carlton Fredericks in his book, *Low Blood Sugar and You.*
14. Martin, Clement G., *Low Blood Sugar, the Hidden Menace of Hypoglycemia*, Arco Publishing Co., N.Y., N.Y., 7th printing, 1976.
15. Weller, Charles, and Boylan, Brian Richard, *How to Live with Hypoglycemia*, Award Books, N.Y., 3rd printing, 1975.

16. Nittler, Alan, "Hypoglycemia," *Let's Live* Magazine, March, 1974, p. 15.
17. Cross, R. J., and Morse, R. E., "Food Facts From Rutgers," July–Sept., 1973, The State University of New Jersey Cooperative Extension Service Report.
18. Yudkin, John, *Sweet and Dangerous*, Peter H. Wyden, N.Y., N.Y., 1972.
19. Abrahamson, E. M., and Pezet, A. W., *Body, Mind and Sugar*, Pyramid Books, N.Y., 1971.
20. Altman, Lawrence K., *The New York Times*, March 15, 1975.
21. Atkins, Robert C., *Dr. Atkins' Diet Revolution*, Bantam Books, Inc., N.Y. 1972.
22. *Lancet*, October 30, 1965.
23. Airola, Paavo, *Cancer: Causes, Prevention and Treatment—The Total Approach*, Health Plus Publishers, P.O. Box 22001, Phoenix, AZ., 1972.
24. McCormick, W. J., "Coronary Thrombosis: A New Concept of Mechanism and Etiology," *Clinical Medicine*, Vol. 4:7, 1957.
25. Pelletier, Omer, the *Journal of the American Medical Association*, April 25, 1969.
26. Egeli, E. S., et al., *American Heart Journal*, Vol. 59, page 527, 1960.
27. Fredericks, Carlton, "Allergy Causes Hypoglycemia," *Prevention*, October, 1974, page 59.
28. Roberts, S. J., the *Journal of the American Geriatrics Society*, June, 1966.
29. *Medical World News*, Oct. 11, 1974.
30. Ershoff, B. H., et al., *Journal of Nutrition*, Vol. 50, page 299, 1953.
31. Hodges, R. E., et al., *Journal of Clinical Investigation*, Vol. 38, page 1421, 1959.
32. Dodger, H., and Seltzer, H. S., *Medical Tribune*, Sept. 12, 1973.
33. Portis, Sydney A., "Life Situations, Emotions, and Hyperinsulinism," the *Journal of the American Medical Association*, Vol. 142: 1281–1286, 1950.
34. Alexander, Franz, "Psychosomatic Medicine," in Proceedings of the Psychotherapy Council, Vol. 2: 41–60, January, 1944.
35. Vascular Research Laboratory Report in *American Medical Association News Release*, June 21, 1965.
36. Visek, Dr. Willard, "Report on Cornell University Research," *Los Angeles Times*, March 29, 1973.

37. Werner, L., and Hambraeus, L., *Acta Societatis Medicorum Upsaliensis*, Vol., 76, No. 5–6.
38. Thomas, W. A., et al., *American Journal of Cardiology*, Jan., 1960, Also, *AMA News Release*, June 21, 1965.
39. Bernstein, D. S., and Wachman, A., Department of Nutrition, Harvard University, "Diet and Osteoporosis," *Lancet*, Vol. 7549, Page 958, 1968.
40. Gerber, Donald A., report in *New York Times*, April 7, 1965.
41. Research by Prof. Ph. Schwartz, and Dr. Ralph Bircher, in *Rejuvenation Secrets From Around the World–that "Work,"* by Dr. Paavo O. Airola, Health Plus Publishers, P.O. Box 22001, Phoenix, AZ., 1974.
42. *A Bircher-Benner Way to Positive Health and Vitality*, Bircher-Benner Verlag, Zurich, Switzerland. Also: Kraut, H. T., Max Planck Institute For Nutrition Research, *Der Wendepunkt*, Vol: 52, page 443, 1975.
43. Eimer, Karl (Klinik Schwenkenbacker), Zeitschriftfu;r, *Ernahrung*, July, 1963.
44. Resolution #80, International Society For Research on Diseases of Civilization and Environment, Belgium.
45. Miller, L. T., et al., *Journal of Nutrition*, September, 1967.
46. Schweigart, H. A., Prof., Dr. Med., *Eiweis, Fette, Herzinfarkt*, Verlag, H. H. Zanner, Mu;nchen.
47. Viktora, Joseph K., et al., *Metabolism, Clinical and Experimental*, Henry M. Stratton, Inc., N.Y., N.Y., Vol. 18, 1969.
48. Jennings, J., "Brewer's Yeast Holds Key to Health," *Prevention*, February, 1974, p. 58.
49. Fredericks, Carlton, "Some Hypoglycemics Need More Starch," *Prevention*, July, 1975, p. 54.
50. Davis, Adelle, *Let's Get Well*, New American Library, Signet paperback, N.Y., 1972, p. 311.
51. Nittler, Alan H., *A New Breed of Doctor*, Pyramid House, N.Y., N.Y., 1972.
52. Barmakian, Richard, *Hypoglycemia, Your Bondage or Freedom*, Altura Health Publishers, Irvine, CA., 1976.
53. Griffin, LaDean, *Is Any Sick Among You?*, Bi-World Publishing Co., Provo, Utah, 1974.
54. Hutchens, Alma R., *Indian Herbology of North America*, 1974.
55. Gray, Bill, M.D., from a communication to the author.
56. Smolyanski, B. L., *Fed. Proceedings*, 22, T1173, 1963.
57. Verzar, F., report to International Congress on Vitamin E, 1955.

INDEX

ABOUT THE AUTHOR

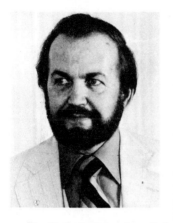

Paavo Airola, Ph.D., N.D., is an internationally recognized nutritionist, naturopathic physician, lecturer, and an award-winning author. He studied nutrition, biochemistry, and biological medicine in Europe and spent many years of research and study in European biological clinics and research centers. He is considered to be the leading authority on biological medicine and wholistic approach to healing in the United States. He lectures extensively, and worldwide, both to professionals and laymen, holding yearly educational seminars for physicians. He has recently lectured at the Stanford University Medical School.

Dr. Airola is the author of eleven widely-read books, notably his two international best-sellers, *Are You Confused?* and *How To Get Well.* The American Academy of Public Affairs issued Dr. Airola the Award of Merit for his book, *There Is A Cure For Arthritis. Are You Confused?* is heralded by many nutritionists, doctors, and critics as "the most important health book ever published," "a must reading for every sincere health seeker."

His comprehensive handbook on natural healing, *How To Get Well,* is the most authoritative and practical manual on biological medicine in print. It outlines complete nutritional, herbal, and other alternative biological therapies for all of our most common ailments and is used as a textbook in several universities and medical schools. It is regarded as a reliable reference manual by doctors, researchers, nutritionists, and students of health, nutrition, and biological medicine.

Dr. Airola's newest book, *Hypoglycemia: A Better Approach,* has revolutionized the concept of and the therapeutic approach to this insidious, complex, and devastating affliction which has assumed epidemic proportions.

Dr. Airola is President of the International Academy of Biological Medicine; a member of the International Naturopathic Association; and a member of the International Society for Research on Civilization Diseases and Environment, the prestigious forum for world-wide research, founded by Dr. Albert Schweitzer. He is listed in *The Directory of International Biography, The Blue Book, The Men of Achievement, Who's Who In American Art,* and *Who's Who in the West.*